Equine En
Transfer

Patrick M. McCue, DVM, PhD, DACT
Edward L. Squires, MS, PhD

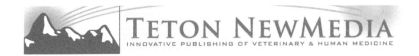

Executive Editor: Carroll C. Cann
Design and Production: www.fiftysixforty.com

Teton NewMedia
P.O. Box 4833
Jackson, WY 83001
1-888-770-3165
tetonnm.com

ISBN# 1-59161-047-8

Printed in the United States

Print Number 5 4 3 2 1

Library of Congress Cataloging-in-Publication Data on file

Preface

The procedures outlined in this manual are based on a combination of basic science, applied research and clinical experience gained from the commercial embryo transfer program at Colorado State University. In addition, techniques and procedures developed in other embryo transfer programs around the world have been incorporated where appropriate.

The goal of this manual is to provide veterinary practitioners and students with general principles and clinical techniques of equine embryo transfer. The authors recognize that there are many ways to successfully collect and transfer equine embryos. It is our estimate that about 90% of procedures in equine embryo transfer performed world-wide are similar if not identical. The other 10% of procedures differ based on geographic location, clinical experience and individual preference and, in some cases unsubstantiated dogma.

It is our hope that experienced practitioners will find useful tips in this manual to enhance embryo collection success or post-transfer pregnancy rates. New graduates and current students may utilize the manual to gain a basic understanding of reproductive principles as well as clinical techniques.

Patrick M. McCue, DVM, PhD, Diplomate American College of Theriogenologists
Colorado State University
Fort Collins, CO USA

Edward Squires, MS, PhD, (hon) Diplomate American College of Theriogenologists
University of Kentucky
Lexington, KY

Acknowledgements

We would like to express our sincere gratitude to Dr. George Seidel, our colleague and University Distinguished Professor, for his expertise and unwavering support of scientific and clinical advancements in embryo transfer.

In addition, we would like to thank the other faculty, staff, residents, graduate students and interns at the Equine Reproduction Laboratory and the Animal Reproduction and Biotechnology Laboratory for their significant contributions over many years.

We are indebted to Drs. Rob Foss and Hunter Ortis from the Equine Medical Services, Columbia, MO, and Drs. Ryan Ferris and Elaine Carnevale from Colorado State University for providing outstanding photographs of *in vivo* and *in vitro* produced equine embryos.

Dr. Patrick McCue
Fort Collins, Colorado

Dr. Edward Squires
Lexington, KY

Table of Contents

Chapter 1

Introduction

Chapter 2

History of Equine Embryo Transfer

Chapter 3

Reproductive Anatomy and Physiology

Chapter 4

Management of the Donor Mare

Chapter 5

Superovulation

Chapter 6
Embryo Collection

Chapter 7
Factors Affecting Embryo Recovery

Chapter 8
Embryo Handling

Chapter 9
Evaluation of Embryos

Chapter 10
Cooled-Transported Embryos

Chapter 11
Cryopreservation of Equine Embryos

Chapter 12
Management of Recipients

Chapter 13
Transfer of Equine Embryos

Chapter 14
Pregnancy Examination after Transfer

Chapter 15
Pregnancy Rates after Transfer

Chapter 16
Factors Affecting Pregnancy Rates

Chapter 17
Disease Transmission

Chapter 18
International Transfer of Embryos

Chapter 19
Related Embryo Technologies

Chapter 20
Future Directions of Equine Embryo Transfer

Appendix I

Appendix II

Index

CHAPTER 1

INTRODUCTION

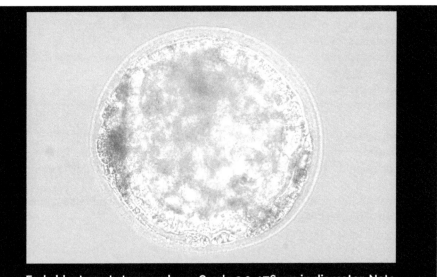

Early blastocyst stage embryo, Grade 2.0, 176 μm in diameter. Note the prominent zona pellucida and developing blastocoele cavity along with a moderate amount of extruded blastomeres. The capsule is visible between the trophoblast layer and the extruded blastomeres.

Principles of Embryo Transfer

Embryo transfer refers to the removal of an embryo from the reproductive tract (i.e. the uterus) of one mare and the transfer of that embryo into the reproductive tract of another mare. Embryo transfer is now a common reproductive procedure in the equine breeding industry. The number of reproductive centers, breeding farms, and veterinary clinics specializing in embryo transfer has increased dramatically in the past 10 years. Advances in collection procedures, transfer techniques, equipment, flush media, embryo shipment and cryopreservation have enhanced the success and therefore the clinical use of embryo transfer in horses.

Potential advantages of embryo transfer include, but are not limited to:
• Valuable mares may have more than one foal per year
• Medical risks associated with pregnancy and parturition are avoided for the donor mare
• Older mares can donate embryos to young recipients
• Mares with reproductive problems can donate embryos to reproductively healthy mares
• Mares with a repeated history of pregnancy loss can donate embryos to recipients
• Mares in athletic competition can donate embryos and remain in performance
• Mares with significant medical or musculoskeletal problems can donate embryos to healthy mares
• Mares that foal late in the season can donate an embryo and still remain open to allow for an early breeding the following year
• Embryos can be cryopreserved and transferred at a later date
• Embryos can be cooled or cryopreserved and transported to a distant location for transfer
• Embryos can be collected from 2 year old donors, which are too young to carry a foal to term themselves
• Embryos can be collected from endangered equids and transferred into domestic mares
• Embryo recovery can be used to evaluate fertility of mares, stallions or semen treatments, providing fertility data 7 or 8 days after ovulation

Breed Regulations

The first foal produced by embryo transfer was born in 1974. Embryo transfer was performed on a somewhat limited basis over the subsequent 30 years due to breed restrictions. Many breed registries either did not allow the procedure or limited the number of foals that could be registered to a given mare per year. The use of embryo transfer in the United States increased dramatically in 2003 when the American Quarter Horse Association (AQHA) eliminated the restriction on the number of foals that could be registered to a given mare in a single year. Previously, the AQHA would allow the registration of only one foal per mare per year. A total of 135,787 foals were registered with the AQHA in 2007, of which approximately 3 % were produced by embryo transfer. The number of foals generated by embryo transfer registered with the AQHA each year from 1980 to 2007 is presented in Figure 1-1.

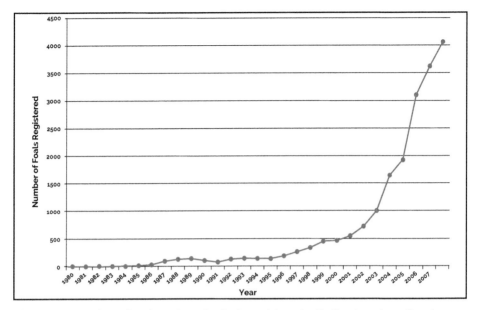

Figure 1-1. Number of embryo transfer foals registered with the American Quarter Horse Association 1980 to 2007.

The American Paint Horse Association and the Arabian Horse Registry of America subsequently followed the lead of the AQHA to not limit the number of foals that could be registered to a specific mare during one season. The American Saddlebred Association has maintained a limit of 4 foals that may be registered to a single mare in one year. The Jockey Club, which is responsible for registration of Thoroughbred horses, does not allow any assisted reproduction procedures, restricting registration of any foals born following artificial insemination, embryo transfer, or other reproductive technologies.

Unequivocally, the largest number of equine embryo transfers being performed in the world today is in Argentinian polo ponies. Embryo transfer programs were initially established in Argentina in the early 1990's. In the largest commercial embryo transfer center, a total of 7,939 pregnancies were obtained from 13,942 collection procedures performed between 1997 and 2010. It has been estimated by the International Embryo Transfer Society that 36,971 embryo collection attempts and 24,491 embryo transfer procedures were performed on horses world-wide in 2009.

Individual breed associations may require notification of the intent to perform embryo transfer and enrollment with the breed registry prior to transfer of an embryo. In most instances, parentage or pedigree must be verified through genetic (DNA) testing of the foal, sire and donor mare. The current regulations regarding embryo transfer and foal registration for several major breed associations are listed in Table 1-1. Owners, breeders and veterinarians are encouraged to contact the appropriate breed associations to verify current regulations, obtain permit applications, and receive registration information.

Table 1-1.
Regulation of embryo transfer by breed association.

Breed Association	Number of Foals Allowed to be Registered per Mare per Year	ET Allowed (yes/no)	Advanced Notification or Permit Required	Parentage (DNA) Verification Required
American Quarter Horse Association (AQHA)	Unlimited	Yes	Yes	Yes
Arabian Horse Association	Unlimited	Yes	Yes	Yes
American Paint Horse Association (APHA)	Unlimited	Yes	Yes	Yes
United States Jockey Club (Thoroughbreds)	1	No	n/a	Yes

There is ongoing debate within breed associations as to the effect of unlimited embryo transfer on the economics, genetics and politics of the horse industry, as well as the reproductive health of the donor mare. Changes in breed registry regulations regarding embryo transfer have certainly allowed for a greater impact of genetics from the dam as compared to previous years. However, acceptance of multiple foals produced by one mare in one season hardly compares with the impact that occurred when approval of artificial insemination and use of transported semen allowed for a tremendous increase in the number of mares bred to an individual stallion within a breeding season.

Potential for Success in Equine Embryo Transfer

In order for an embryo transfer program to be successful, management of the donor mare and recipient mare must be optimal and the techniques of embryo collection and transfer must be well understood. Ultimately, the success of an embryo transfer program can be measured by a simple formula:

ET Pregnancy Rate per Cycle = Embryo Collection Rate (%) x Transfer Pregnancy Rate (%)

Mares usually spontaneously ovulate only one follicle per cycle. In the absence of effective hormones for superovulation, embryo collection attempts are therefore based on one potential embryo per cycle. In reality, the overall embryo collection rate is approximately 50 to 65% per cycle, with variability depending on the inherent fertility of the mare and stallion, type of semen used and many other factors. Pregnancy rate after transfer is approximately 70 to 90%, with considerable variability depending on the experience of the transfer technician, quality of the embryo, and factors associated with the recipient mare. Consequently, the range of

4

predicted success (i.e. a pregnant recipient mare) for one embryo transfer cycle is 35 to 59 % per cycle.

ET Pregnancy Rate per Cycle   = (50-65%) x (70-90%)
                                = 35 to 59%

In addition, approximately 8 to 10 % of pregnancies are lost between initial detection of pregnancy (i.e. day 12 to 16) and the expected due date. The rate of pregnancy loss is similar between embryo transfer recipient mares and mares bred to carry their own pregnancy.

Horse owners should be apprised of the factors that go into embryo transfer and provided realistic expectations for success, which is establishment of pregnancy in a recipient mare and birth of a live foal. These expectations should be based on the individual donor mare and stallion.

The goal of this Manual is to provide veterinarians, horse owners, breeding managers, and students with a solid foundation in the principles, techniques and expectations for equine embryo transfer.

Recommended Reading

Riera F. General techniques and organization of large commercial embryo transfer programs. Clinical Theriogenology 2011; 3: 318-324.

Squires EL, Seidel Jr., GE. Collection and transfer of equine embryos. Colorado State University Animal Reproduction and Biotechnology Laboratory Bulletin No. 8, 1995; 64 pp.

Squires EL, Carnevale EM, McCue PM, Bruemmer JE. Embryo technologies in the horse. Theriogenology 2003; 59:151-170.

Stout TAE. Equine embryo transfer: review of developing potential. Equine Veterinary Journal 2006; 38:467-478.

CHAPTER 2

HISTORY OF EQUINE EMBRYO TRANSFER

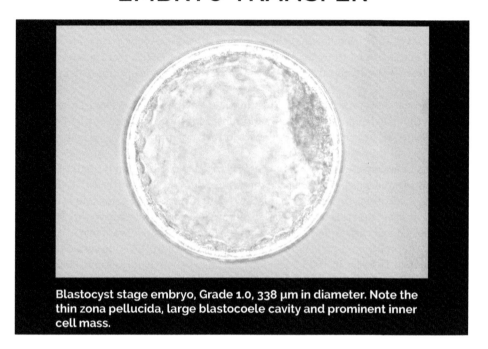

Blastocyst stage embryo, Grade 1.0, 338 µm in diameter. Note the thin zona pellucida, large blastocoele cavity and prominent inner cell mass.

Embryo Transfer in Domestic Animals

The first successful production of live young by embryo transfer was performed in rabbits in 1890. Rabbits were used extensively as research models in the field of embryology throughout the end of the 19th century and the early decades of the 20th century. Successful transfers of rat and mouse embryos were initially performed in the 1930's. Early efforts in embryo biology of large animal species also began in this decade.

The first successful transfers of sheep, pig and cattle embryos were reported in the early 1950's. Surgical transfer of embryos into the uterus of the recipient was the most successful technique used in the early days of large animal embryo transfer. Birth of calves and pigs following nonsurgical, transcervical embryo transfer were reported in the 1960's. However, it was not until the mid-1970's that transcervical embryo transfer replaced surgical embryo transfer as a routine procedure in cattle.

In 1972 researchers reported the birth of live mouse offspring that were derived from embryos that had been frozen, thawed and subsequently transferred. A year later came a report of the first calf born following transfer of a frozen-thawed embryo.

Transport of embryos over long distances was first accomplished in the early 1970's by placing pig and sheep embryos into the oviducts of rabbits, which were used as biological incubators. The 1970's was also an era of micromanipulation and early attempts at *in vitro* fertilization. The first calf produced from an embryo that had been biopsied and the sex determined from the biopsy specimen was born in 1975. The first calf produced from *in vitro* fertilization was born in 1981. This was followed by the birth of **IVF** pigs in 1983 and lambs in 1984. The birth of the lamb 'Dolly', the first animal born following nuclear transfer or cloning, occurred in 1986.

History of Equine Embryo Transfer

The era of equine embryo transfer began in 1972 with a report of reciprocal inter-species transfer of horse, donkey, mule or hinny zygotes collected from and transferred back into mares or donkeys. This was followed in 1974 by the birth of a live horse foal produced by embryo transfer. Initially, equine embryos were transferred immediately after collection until techniques and culture media for successful cooling and short-term storage were described in the late 1980's. This opened up new clinical opportunities in which embryos were collected at one site, cooled and shipped to a specialized transfer center often located a long distance away.

Successful cryopreservation of an equine embryo that resulted in a live foal was first reported in 1982. A variety of techniques for embryo cryopreservation have been described, with the most successful involving either slow freezing or vitrification (ultrarapid freezing) of small (< 300 μm) embryos. Advanced assisted reproduction technologies such as oocyte transfer **(OT)**, intracytoplasmic sperm injection **(ICSI)**, and nuclear transfer **(NT)** were introduced to the equine breeding industry in the late 1990's and early 2000's (Table 2-1).

Concepts and techniques initially developed in other species have been subsequently used by equine reproduction specialists over the decades. The state-of-the-art of

Table 2-1.
Milestones Related to Equine Embryo Transfer

Year	Milestone	Reference
1966	Recognition that unfertilized equine oocytes are retained in oviduct	Van Niekerk and Gerneke, 1966
1972	Birth of the first equid offspring by embryo transfer	Allen and Rowson, 1972
1974	Birth of the first foal produced by embryo transfer	Oguri and Tsutsumi, 1974
1974	First report of superovulation of mares	Douglas et al., 1974
1975	First non-surgical equine embryo transfer	Allen and Rowson, 1975
1976	Long-distance transport of equine embryos in a rabbit reported	Allen et al., 1976
1982	Capsule of the equine embryo first described	Flood et al., 1982
1982	Foal born following transfer of a frozen-thawed embryo	Yamamoto et al., 1982
1984	Production of twins following bisection of an equine embryo	Allen and Pashen, 1984; Slade et al., 1984
1985	International transport of equine embryos	Boyle et al., 1985
1985	Pregnancies established after transfer of embryos into ovariectomized mares	Hinrichs et al., 1985
1985	Successful transfer of zebra embryo into domestic horse mare	Bennett and Foster, 1985
1985	Successful transfer of Przewalski horse embryo into domestic horse mare	Kydd et al., 1985
1987	Technique developed for successful cooling of equine embryos	Carnevale et al., 1987
1988	Birth of first foal following oocyte transfer	McKinnon et al., 1988
1989	First embryo produced from *in vitro* matured equine oocytes	Zhang et al., 1989
1991	Birth of first foal produced by *in vitro* fertilization	Palmer et al., 1991

Table 2-1. Continued

Year	Milestone	Reference
1991	Recognition that PGE2 production by embryo facilitates oviductal transport	Weber et al., 1991
1992	Superovulation of mares by immunization against inhibin	McCue et al., 1992; McKinnon et al., 1992
1996	First foal produced from intra-cytoplasmic sperm injection (ICSI)	Squires et al., 1996
1997	Biopsy of equine embryos first reported	Huhtinen et al., 1997
1999	Birth of foal after oocyte transfer into nonovulating, hormone-treated recipient mare	Hinrichs et al., 1999
2000	First pregnancy from flow-sorted (sexed) stallion spermatozoa	Schmid et al., 2000
2002	First foals born following transfer of vitrified oocytes	Maclellan et al., 2002
2003	Birth of a mule foal produced by cloning	Woods et al., 2003
2003	Birth of first horse foal produced by cloning	Galli et al., 2003
2003	Pregnancies obtained from oocytes collected from euthanized mares	Carnevale et al., 2003
2003	Superovulation of mares with purified equine FSH	Niswender et al., 2003
2004	Development of recombinant equine FSH	Roser et al., 2004
2010	Foal born after transfer of biopsied, vitrified embryo	Troedsson et al., 2010
2011	Cryopreservation of expanded equine blastocysts	Choi et al., 2011
2013	Autogenous transfer of ICSI-produced embryos	Carnevale et al., 2013

equine embryo transfer at the present time includes superovulation, transfer of fresh or cooled-transported embryos, and vitrification of embryos. Embryos are also being produced in a limited number of specialized research laboratories and private reproduction centers by oocyte collection, intracytoplasmic sperm injection, and nuclear transfer. Equine embryos have also been biopsied for determination of genetic sex and subsequently cryopreserved or transferred into recipient mares with success.

Research is the basis for advancement of any scientific discipline and continued research in the areas of cryopreservation, genetic testing and superovulation will provide for advancement of the science and clinical application of equine embryo transfer.

Recommended Reading

Allen WR, Rowson LEA. Transfer of ova between horses and donkeys. In: Proc., 7th Int. Congress on Animal Reproduction and Artificial Insemination. 6-9 June 1972, Munich. 1972; p. 484-487.

Allen WR, Rowson LEA. Surgical and non-surgical egg transfer in horses. J. Reprod. Fertil. Suppl. 1975;23:525-530.

Allen WR, Stewart F, Trounson AO, Tischner M, Bielanski W. Viability of horse embryos after storage and long-distance transport in the rabbit. J Reprod Fertil 1976; 47:387-390.

Allen WR, Pashen RL. Production of monozygotic (identical) horse twins by embryo micromanipulation. J Reprod Fertil 1984; 71:607-613.

Bennett SD, Foster WR. Successful transfer of a zebra embryo to a domestic horse. Equine Vet. J. 1985; 3: 78-79.

Betteridge KJ. A history of farm animal embryo transfer and some associated techniques. Animal Reproduction Science 2003; 79:203-244.

Boyle MS, Allen WR, Tischner M, Czlonkowska M. Storage and international transport of horse embryos in liquid nitrogen. Equine Vet. J. Suppl. 1985; 36-39.

Carnevale EM, Squires EL, Cook VM, Seidel Jr., GE, Jasko DJ. Comparison of Ham's F-10 with CO_2 or Hepes buffer for the 24 hr storage of equine embryos at 5° C. J Anim Sci 1987; 65:1775-1781.

Carnevale EM, Maclellan LJ, Coutinho da Silva MA, Squires EL. Pregnancies attained after collection and transfer of oocytes from ovaries of five euthanized mares. J Amer Vet Med Assoc 2003; 222:60-62.

Carnevale EM, Rossini JB, Rodriguez J, Bresnahan DR, Stokes JE Autogenous transfers of intracytoplasmic sperm injection-produced equine embryos in oocyte donor uteri. Annual Convention American Association of Equine Practitioners 2013; 59; 200-203.

Choi YH, Velez IC. Riera FL, Roldan JE, Hartman DL, Bliss SB, Blanchard TL, Hayden SS, Hinrichs K. Successful cryopreservation of expanded equine blastocytes. Theriogenology 2011; 76: 143-152.

Douglas RH, Nuti L, Ginther OJ. Induction of ovulation and multiple ovulation in seasonally anovulatory mares with equine pituitary fractions. Theriogenology 1974; 2:133-142.

Flood PF, Betteridge KJ, Diocee MS. Transmission electron microscopy of horse embryos three to 16 days after ovulation. J Reprod Fertil, Suppl. 1982; 32:319-327.

Galli C, Lagutina, Crotti G, Colleoni S, Turini P, Ponderato N, Duchi R, Lazzari G. A cloned horse born to its dam twin. Nature 2003; 424:635.

Hinrichs K, Sertich PL, Cummings MR, Kenney RM. Pregnancy in ovariectomized mares achieved by embryo transfer: a preliminary study. Equine Veterinary Journal 1985; 17(S3): 74-75.

Hinrichs K. Assisted reproduction techniques in the horse. Reprod Fertil Develop 2013; 25: 80-93.

Hinrichs K, Provost PJ, Torello EM. Birth of a foal after oocyte transfer to a nonovulating, hormone-treated recipient mare. Theriogenology 1999; 51: 1251-1258.

Huhtinen M, Peippo J, Bredbacka P. Successful transfer of biopsied equine embryos. Theriogenology 1997; 48: 361-367.

Kydd J, Boyle MS, Allen WR, Shephard A, Summers PM. Transfer of exotic equine embryos to domestic horses and donkeys. Equine Vet J. 1985; 3: 80-83.

Maclellan LJ, Carnevale EM, Coutinho da Silva MA, Scoggin CF, Bruemmer JE, Squires EL. Pregnancies from vitrified equine oocytes collected from superstimulated and non-stimulated mares. Theriogenology 2002; 58:911–919.

McCue PM, Carney NJ, Hughes JP, Rivier J, Vale W, Lasley BL. Ovulation and embryo recovery rates following immunization of mares against an inhibin alpha-subunit. Equine Vet J 1992; 38: 823-831.

McKinnon AO, Brown RW, Pashen RL, Greenwood PE, Vassey JR. Increased ovulation rates in mares after immunization against recombinant bovine inhibin alpha-subunit. Equine Vet J 1992; 24: 144-146.

McKinnon AO, Carnevale, Squires EL, Voss JL, Seidel Jr, GE. Heterogenous and xenogenous fertilization of in vivo matured equine oocytes. J Equine Vet Sci 1988; 8:143-147.

Niswinder KD, Alvarenga MA, McCue PM, Hardy QP, Squires EL. Superovulation in cycling mares using equine follicle stimulating hormone (eFSH). J Equine Vet Sci 2003; 23: 497-500.

Palmer E, Bezard J, Magistrini M, Duchamp G. In vitro fertilization in the horse: a retrospective study. J Reprod Fertil, Suppl 1991; 44:375-384.

Oguri N, Tsutsumi Y. Non-surgical egg transfer in mares. J Reprod Fertil 1974; 41:313-320.

Roser JF, Jablonka-Shariff A, Daphna-Iken D, Boime I. Expression and bioactivity of single chain recombinant equine luteinizing hormone (LH) and follicle stimulating hormone (FSH). In: Proceedings of the 15th International Congress on Animal Reproduction; Porto Seguro, Brazil; August 8-12, 2004; 572.

Schmid RL, Kato H, Herickhoff LA, Schenk JL, McCue PM, Chung YG, Squires EL. Effects of follicular fluid or progesterone on in vitro maturation of equine oocytes before intracytoplasmic sperm injection with non-sorted and sex-sorted spermatozoa. J Reprod Fert 2000; 56:519–525.

Slade NP, Williams TJ, Squires EL, Seidel Jr., GE. Production of identical twin pregnancies by microsurgical bisection of equine embryos. Proc 10th Int Congr Anim Reprod Artificial Insemination. 1984; 10:241.

Squires EL, Wilson JM, Kato H, Blaszczyk A. A pregnancy after intracytoplasmic sperm injection into equine oocytes matured in vitro. Theriogenology 1996; 45:306.

Van Niekerk CH, Gerneke WH. Persistence and parthenogenetic cleavage of tubal ova in the mare. Onderstepoort J Vet Res 1966; 33:195-232.

Weber JA, Freeman DA, Vanderwall DK, Woods GL. Prostaglandin E2 secretion by oviductal transport-stage equine embryos. Biol Reprod 1991; 45:540-543.

Woods GL, White KL, Vanderwall DK, Li GP, Aston KL, Bunch TD, Meerdo LN, Pate BJ. A mule cloned from fetal cells by nuclear transfer. Science 2003; 301:1063.

Yamamoto Y, Oguri N, Tsutsumi Y, Hachinohe Y. Experiments in the freezing and storage of equine embryos. J Reprod Fertil, Suppl 1982; 32:399-403.

Zhang JJ, Boyle MS, Allen WR, Galli C. Recent studies on *in vivo* fertilization of in vitro matured horse oocytes. Equine Vet Journal, 1989; Supplement 8:101-104.

CHAPTER 3

REPRODUCTIVE ANATOMY AND PHYSIOLOGY

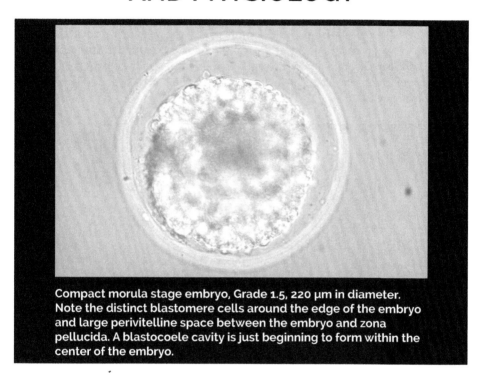

Compact morula stage embryo, Grade 1.5, 220 µm in diameter. Note the distinct blastomere cells around the edge of the embryo and large perivitelline space between the embryo and zona pellucida. A blastocoele cavity is just beginning to form within the center of the embryo.

Introduction

It is important to have an understanding of normal reproductive anatomy and physiology of the mare in order to successfully perform reproductive procedures such as artificial insemination, embryo collection and embryo transfer. The goal of this chapter is to review salient concepts of reproductive anatomy, reproductive physiology, and early embryonic development.

Reproductive Anatomy

The equine ovary is suspended in the dorso-lateral abdomen by a portion of the broad ligament called the mesovarium. A thick connective tissue membrane called the tunica albuginea covers a majority of the ovary. The only exception is the ovulation fossa, a prominent depression on the ventral border of the equine ovary through which all ovulations take place. The ovulation fossa is lined by a layer of cells termed the germinal epithelium (Figure 3-1).

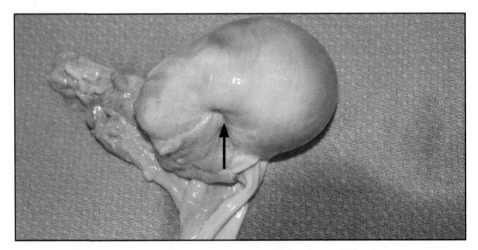

Figure 3-1. Equine ovary. Note the prominent ovulation fossa (arrow).

Females do not produce new gametes after birth. Consequently, a filly foal is born with a full complement of oocytes within her ovaries. Puberty is reached at approximately 16 to 20 months of age. Thereafter, during the physiologic breeding season equine ovaries will contain follicles and luteal structures in various stages of development and regression. The dominant follicle increases in diameter by 3 to 5 mm per day during estrus. Preovulatory follicles in the mare are approximately 40 to 45 mm in diameter. The size of the preovulatory follicle is breed dependent, with Quarter Horse and Arabian breeds ovulating follicles 35 to 45 mm in diameter, Thoroughbred and Standardbred mares typically ovulating follicles 40 to 50 mm in diameter, Warmblood mares ovulating follicles 45 to 55 mm in diameter, and draft mares ovulating follicles 50 to 60 mm in diameter.

At ovulation, the follicle ruptures into the ovulation fossa releasing follicular fluid and the oocyte. The collapsed follicle eventually fills with blood forming the corpus hemorrhagicum **(CH)**. The corpus luteum **(CL)** forms as luteinized granulosa and theca cells from the follicular wall invade into the blood clot. The mature corpus luteum of the mare is 20 to 30 mm in diameter and is contained within the tissue of the ovary and therefore cannot be detected easily by transrectal palpation. The corpus albicans **(CA)** is the inactive remnant of the corpus luteum after prostaglandin-induced luteolysis.

The oviduct collects the oocyte after ovulation and the ampullary region of the oviduct is the site of fertilization. The oviduct is subdivided into 3 regions, the infundibulum, ampulla and isthmus. The infundibulum is the funnel-shaped end of the oviduct adjacent to the ovary. Irregular finger-like processes called fimbria are located at the cranial border of the infundibulum. In the mare the infundibulum covers the ovulation fossa and facilitates pickup and transport of the oocyte into the oviduct. The ampulla is the central portion of the oviduct and is located between the infundibulum and the isthmus. The isthmus is the caudal segment of the oviduct that is attached to the tip of the uterine horn. The opening of the oviduct into uterus is the uterotubular junction.

The uterus is designed to support and protect the early developing embryo, provide structural and functional support for the placenta, and eventually cause contractions sufficient for expulsion of the fetus at parturition. Mares have a 'Y' shaped uterus, with two uterine horns of medium length and a relatively short uterine body.

The uterus is suspended in the caudal abdomen of the mare by a portion of the broad ligament called the mesometrium. A major blood vessel supplying the uterus, the middle uterine artery, traverses through the broad ligament (Figure 3-2).

The outer surface layer of the uterus is called the serosa. The myometrium, or muscular layer, is comprised of two layers of smooth muscle; an inner circular layer and an outer longitudinal layer. The endometrium, or internal lining of the uterus, contains glands which produce substances, commonly referred to as histiotroph or, "uterine milk", which provides nutrition to the early embryo. The endometrium is also the surface to which the placenta will eventually attach via structures called microcotyledons.

The cervix is a thick-walled tubular muscle located between the uterus and the vagina. In the mare, the cervix is approximately 7.5 to 10 cm (3" to 4") in length. The external os of the cervix protrudes about 1 to 2 cm into the vagina in the mare. Numerous small longitudinal folds of mucous membrane line the lumen of the cervix or cervical canal. These cervical folds are continuous with the folds of the endometrium.

Tone and character of the cervix change dramatically during the different stages of the estrous cycle in response to the prevailing ovarian steroid hormone. In estrus, the cervix is soft, relaxed, and opens in response to elevated levels of estradiol and an absence of progesterone. This allows semen to pass through the cervical canal into the uterine lumen during natural breeding and allows for clearance of dead spermatozoa, inflammatory cells and fluid by uterine contractions after breeding.

In diestrus, the increase in progesterone causes the cervix to close and increase in tone. The cervix functions as a major physical barrier, in addition to the vulva and vestibulo-vaginal fold to prevent bacteria and other microorganisms from ascending into the uterus.

The vagina is a muscular structure that extends from the vestibular-vaginal fold cranially to the cervix. The hymen is a membranous fold located at the vestibular-vaginal junction. A hymen may be present in maiden mares and may vary from a thin band to an imperforate structure that completely occludes the external orifice

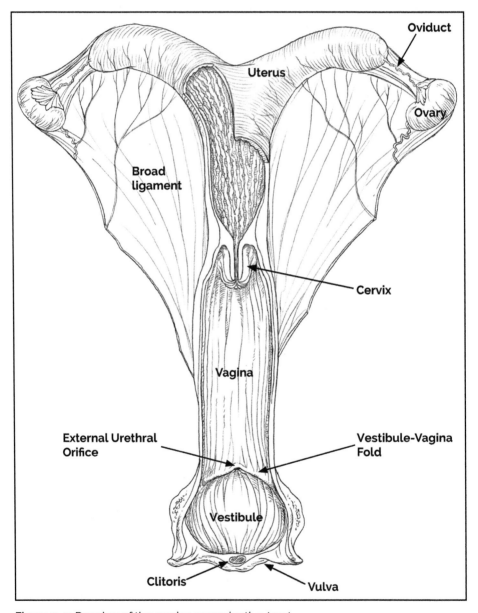

Figure 3-2. Drawing of the equine reproductive tract.

of the vagina. The hymen is a remnant of tissue that sometimes remains where the paramesonephric ducts joined the urogenital sinus in embryonic development.

The vestibule is the portion of the female reproductive tract that lies between the vulva and the vagina. The cranial border of the vestibule is the vestibular-vaginal fold or transverse fold. The external urethral orifice is located caudal to the transverse fold on the ventral surface of the vestibule and is the entrance to the urinary bladder.

The vulva is the caudal termination of the genital tract and is comprised of paired labia, dorsal and ventral commissures and the clitoris. The labia or lips of the vulva are homologous to the scrotum of the male and the clitoris is homologous to the glans penis of the male.

The vulva and the surrounding area is referred to as the perineal area or perineum. The ideal perineal conformation in mares has the vulva situated in a vertical position, with approximately two-thirds of the vulva located below the pelvic brim (Figure 3-3). Tilting or angling of the dorsal aspect of the vulva cranially and poor muscular tone to the vulva predispose the mare to ascending uterine infections.

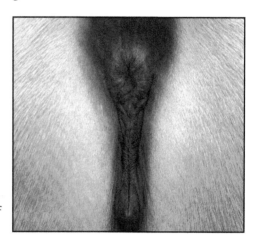

Figure 3-3. Normal perineal anatomy of a mare.

Reproductive Physiology
Seasonality and the Transition Period
The natural or physiologic breeding season of horses extends from April to October in the Northern Hemisphere. Mares are polyestrus in that they exhibit repeated estrous cycles during the breeding season.

Seasonal anestrus is often subdivided into deep anestrus and transition (shallow anestrus) periods depending on the amount of follicular activity present. Deep anestrus is characterized by minimal ovarian follicular development (i.e. follicles < 20 mm in diameter). The behavior of mares in deep anestrus may range from receptive (teasing in), to indifferent (passive), to unreceptive (teasing out) reflecting a general absence of influence from ovarian steroid hormones.

A progressive increase in the duration of the ambient photoperiod in the spring stimulates ovarian function. This is mediated by a change in melatonin production from the pineal gland in response to day length. Melatonin is released during the hours of darkness and a decrease in the duration of melatonin exposure in the spring leads to an increase in GnRH production and subsequently an increase in pituitary gonadotropin secretion and stimulation of ovarian follicular development.

From a practical standpoint, the onset of transition in mares occurs when the first developing follicle of the season reaches 20 to 25 mm in diameter. Mares may exhibit one wave or multiple waves of follicular growth and regression during the transition period. The total number of follicles present on each ovary increases during the transition, and ultrasound examination classically reveals a "grape-like" cluster of small to medium sized follicles. The transition period may last for 50 to 70 days or more prior to the first ovulation of the season. Once a mare has ovulated, she will generally continue to cycle at regular intervals. Behaviorally, transitional mares may display prolonged or irregular periods of estrus in response to estrogens produced by the developing follicles.

The mean calendar date of the first spontaneous ovulation of the year in anestrous mares maintained under ambient light conditions in North America ranges from the middle of March to early May.

Physiologic Breeding Season

Mares ovulate at approximately 21 day intervals throughout the breeding season. The equine estrous cycle can be divided into 2 phases, based on sexual receptivity. Estrus refers to the period during which mares are receptive to advances of the stallion (Figure 3-4). Behavioral estrus typically lasts 5-7 days and is stimulated by increasing levels of the hormone estradiol produced by the developing dominant follicle and

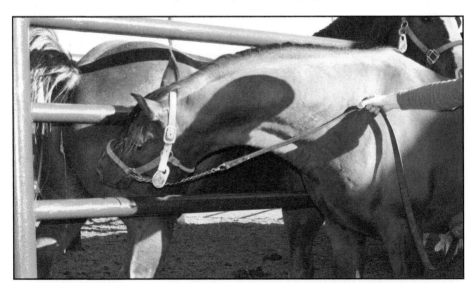

Figure 3-4. A mare in estrus (teasing in heat). Note the base-wide stance and elevated tail.

the absence of progesterone. Diestrus refers to the period during which mares reject advances of the stallion (Figure 3-5). Progesterone production by the corpus luteum controls the behavioral responses of the mare during the 14 to 16 day diestrous period.

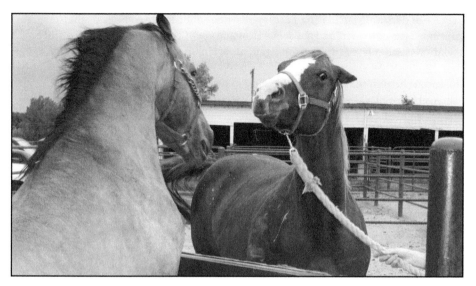

Figure 3-5. A mare (right) in diestrus (teasing out of heat) being teased by a stallion (left).

Mares utilize an active process of follicular selection to limit the number of ovulations in most estrous cycles to one. The mechanism of follicle selection involves a complex, closely associated interaction between pituitary gonadotropins and ovarian hormones. The major or primary follicular wave of the equine estrous cycle, or the wave that ends with ovulation during estrus, originates in diestrus approximately 7 to 8 days after ovulation when a cohort of follicles emerge from a pool of smaller follicles over a period of several days. After emergence, follicles in the wave go through a common-growth phase for approximately 6-7 days during which all follicles increase in size at approximately the same rate (3 mm/day). Deviation occurs at the end of the common-growth phase and represents the point at which the future dominant follicle continues to develop and smaller subordinate follicles regress.

Follicle stimulating hormone **(FSH)** produced by the anterior pituitary gland provides the drive for emergence and initial growth. All of the follicles in the follicular wave require FSH for initial growth and development. The future dominant follicle usually emerges approximately 1 day earlier than the other follicles in the wave. Consequently, this follicle is slightly larger than the other follicles in the cohort at the end of the common-growth phase. Circulating levels of FSH peak when the largest follicle is approximately 13 mm in diameter. Inhibin and estradiol produced by the larger follicles within the wave cause a reduction in FSH secretion (Figure 3-6). Follicle deviation takes place approximately 3 days after the FSH peak as levels of FSH are declining and the diameter of the largest follicle is approximately 22 to 25 mm. The process of deviation represents selection against future development of subordinate follicles by factors produced by the dominant follicle. The developing dominant follicle becomes increasingly responsive to FSH and luteinizing hormone **(LH)** as compared to other (smaller) follicles in the wave, due in part to an increase in the number of gonadotropin receptors in the dominant follicle stimulated by elevated intrafollicular estradiol levels. Consequently, the larger follicle continues to develop in the face of declining circulating FSH levels while subordinate follicles begin to regress. Continued development and subsequent ovulation of the dominant follicle after deviation is stimulated by the prolonged elevation or surge of LH.

The corpus luteum that forms after ovulation produces progesterone which is responsible for blocking the expression of behavioral estrus, altering the secretion and development of endometrial glands, closure of the cervix and a variety of other physiologic processes. Progesterone concentration at the time of ovulation is low (< 0.5 ng/ml). Levels begin to increase above 1.0 ng/ml 1 to 2 days after ovulation as

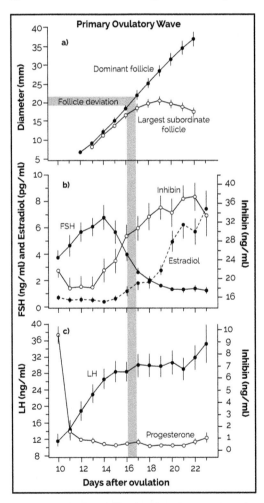

Figure 3-6. Hormone profiles during follicular development and estrus in mares (From DR Bergfelt and GP Adams. Ovulation and corpus luteum development. In: JC Samper, JF Pycock and AO McKinnon. Current Therapy in Equine Reproduction, Saunders Elsevier, St. Louis, 2007, pp. 1-13.).

the corpus luteum forms (Figure 3-7). Consequently, mares usually go out of heat 1 to 2 days after ovulation. Progesterone levels peak at approximately day 5 and slowly decline until day 12 to 14 after ovulation. In the non-pregnant mare, pulsatile secretion of prostaglandins from the endometrium causes destruction of the corpus luteum or luteolysis. This provides the mare an opportunity to return to estrus and cycle again.

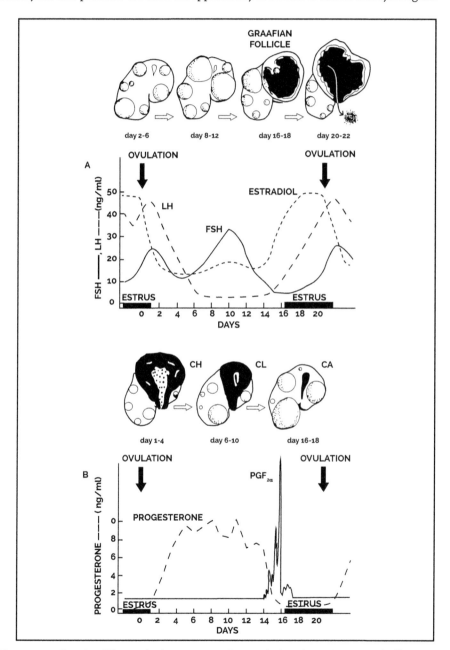

Figure 3-7. Graph of the major hormone patterns during the estrous cycle (from PF Daels and JP Hughes. The Normal Estrous Cycle. In: AO McKinnon and JL Voss (eds). Equine Reproduction, Williams and Wilkins, Baltimore, 1993, pp 121-132.).

Physiology of Early Pregnancy

Embryo biology of the horse has several unique features not found in other domestic animals. Mares ovulate one or occasionally two or more follicles near the end of estrus. The oocytes are "collected" by the infundibulum of the oviduct and transported distally toward the uterus. If the mare has been bred or inseminated, spermatozoa migrate proximally up the oviduct toward the newly ovulated oocyte(s) and fertilization occurs in the ampullary region of the oviduct. Although mares are usually bred with 500 million to several billion spermatozoa, only a few thousand sperm actually make it into the oviduct.

Spermatozoa undergo a series of changes in the mare reproductive tract, a process called capacitation, in order to gain the ability to fertilize an oocyte. Capacitated sperm bind to specific proteins in the zona pellucida of the oocyte. Binding to the oocyte triggers an event in the sperm termed the acrosome reaction, in which enzymes present in the acrosomal cap located on the head of the sperm are released. These enzymes enable the sperm to penetrate through the zona pellucida. The plasma membranes of the sperm and egg subsequently fuse and the sperm is eventually engulfed into the oocyte. The oocyte then undergoes the cortical reaction which prevents additional sperm from penetrating. Fusion of the pronuclei of the sperm and egg, which contain DNA from the stallion and mare, respectively, results in formation of the genetic blueprint of the new embryo (Figure 3-8).

The newly formed embryo begins a series of cleavage divisions in which the single-celled zygote divides into 2 cells, then 4 cells, etc. The embryo continues to develop as it travels distally within the oviduct. Horses are unique among domestic animals in that only fertilized eggs or embryos are transported into the uterus. Equine embryos produce a hormone called prostaglandin E_2 **(PGE$_2$)** which causes relaxation of the circular muscle and contraction of the longitudinal muscle of the distal oviductal wall. PGE_2 allows the embryo to traverse through the isthmus region of the oviduct and eventually pass through the utero-tubular junction **(UTJ)** into the uterus. Unfertilized oocytes do not produce PGE_2 and are consequently retained in the oviduct near the ampulla-isthmus junction and eventually degenerate. Occasionally an unfertilized oocyte will be recovered from the uterus during an

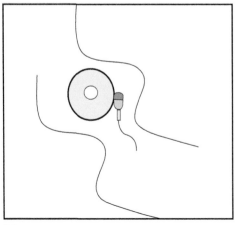

Figure 3-8. Sperm-oocyte interaction in the equine oviduct.

embryo flush procedure if it follows an embryo producing PGE$_2$ through the oviduct.

Equine embryos enter the uterus through a narrow passage called the utero-tubular junction approximately 130 to 142 hours (5.5 to 6.5 days) after ovulation. At this time most equine embryos are in either the morula or early blastocyst stage of development.

A unique glycoprotein investment called the "capsule" is produced by secretions from trophoblast cells of the equine embryo beginning approximately 5 to 6 days after ovulation. Initially the capsule is located between the trophoblast layer and the zona pellucida. The zona pellucida thins and is eventually shed as the embryo develops and expands. Subsequently, the capsule becomes the outermost investment surrounding the embryo. The exact function(s) of the capsule are not well understood. The capsule may provide physical protection to the spherical embryo and help facilitate migration of the embryo throughout the uterus which is critical for maternal recognition of pregnancy. Interestingly, a capsule does not form in equine embryos produced *in vitro*.

Contractions of the uterine musculature cause the equine embryo to be transported throughout the uterus multiple times per day. During this mobility phase, the embryo signals the endometrium that a pregnancy is present. A pregnancy recognition factor has been identified in cattle, sheep, pigs and several other species, but the signal has yet to be identified in the horse. This embryo-uterus interaction, called maternal recognition of pregnancy, is a key component of pregnancy maintenance in the mare.

Failure of the embryo to produce a sufficient signal or failure of the uterus to recognize the signal will result in the release of prostaglandins (**PGF$_{2\alpha}$**) from the endometrium. Prostaglandins travel through the blood stream and cause regression of the corpus luteum. Regression of the CL results in a cessation of progesterone production and loss of any pregnancy that may be present. The window for maternal recognition of pregnancy in the mare is approximately 12 to 16 days after ovulation. Embryo migration ceases at approximately 16 to 17 days after ovulation and the embryo is then "fixed" in position at the base of one uterine horn.

Recommended Reading

Bergfelt DR. Anatomy and physiology of the mare. In: Samper JC (Ed), Equine Breeding Management and Artificial Insemination, Second Edition; Saunders Elsevier, St. Louis, 2009; pp.113-131.

Evans TJ, Constantinescu GM, Ganjam VK. Clinical reproductive anatomy and physiology of the mare. In: Younquist RS and Threlfall WR (Eds). Current Therapy in Large Animal Theriogenology, vol. 2; Saunders Elsevier, St. Louis, 2007; pp.47-67.

Kainer RA. Internal reproductive anatomy. In: McKinnon AO, Squires EL, Vaala WE, Varner DD (Eds). Equine Reproduction, Second Edition; Wiley-Blackwell, Ames, Iowa; 2011; pp. 1582-1600.

Löfstedt RM. Diestrus. In: McKinnon AO, Squires EL, Vaala WE, Varner DD (Eds). Equine Reproduction, Second Edition; Wiley-Blackwell, Ames, Iowa; 2011; pp. 1728-1731.

McCue PM, Scoggin CF, Lindholm ARG. Estrus. In: McKinnon AO, Squires EL, Vaala WE, Varner DD (Eds). Equine Reproduction, Second Edition; Wiley-Blackwell, Ames, Iowa; 2011; pp. 1716-1727.

CHAPTER 4

MANAGEMENT OF
THE DONOR MARE

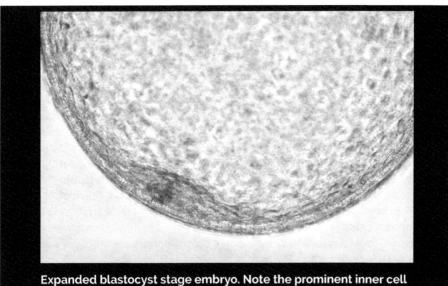

Expanded blastocyst stage embryo. Note the prominent inner cell mass protruding into the blastocoele cavity from the trophoblast layer.

Selection of the Donor Mare

The best embryo donors are reproductively healthy mares in good body condition and free of stress and disease. In general, optimal health and breeding management of the donor mare is essential for embryo collection success. Routine management should include nutrition, dental care, foot care, vaccination, deworming, housing and exercise.

Embryo collection is not often very efficient in young mares, old mares or mares with a history of subfertility or infertility. Embryo collection efficiency is low in mares early in their 2-year-old year and improves later that season. Embryo collection rates are also lower in older mares (i.e. greater than 15 years of age) due to decreased oocyte quality and age related effects on uterine health. In addition, pregnancy loss rates may be higher in recipients carrying embryos from older donor mares.

Seasonal Reproductive Management

Donor mares should be maintained under an artificial photoperiod to provide 16 hours of light and allow 8 hours of darkness per day to advance the first ovulation of the year. Approximately 60 days of a stimulatory artificial photoperiod are required to induce ovulation. Light therapy should be instituted by approximately December 1 (North America) to stimulate follicular development and ovulation by early February. A minimum of 10 foot-candles (approximately 100 lux) beginning at dusk for 3 or more hours are required to provide sufficient light to have a biological effect. Incandescent or fluorescent lights are both effective. A convenient strategy is to set a timer to turn lights on just prior to dusk and turn lights off at approximately 11:00 pm. Exposure to artificial photoperiod should continue until late March or early April in North America, after which the light therapy can safely be discontinued and mares will continue to cycle.

Reproductive Evaluation of Donor Mares

Ideally, a reproductive evaluation should be performed on donor mares at the end of the breeding season or in the early fall to identify and correct potential reproductive problems. The donor mare should also be examined prior to or at the beginning of the breeding season. The examination should include:
• Physical examination
• Perineal examination
• Palpation and ultrasound examination per rectum
• Uterine culture
• Uterine cytology

Additional procedures may include:
• Vaginal speculum examination
• Endometrial biopsy

The goals of the examination are to determine if the mare is in adequate physical condition, identify potential medical issues, monitor ovarian status, and evaluate uterine health.

Reproductive Management of Donor Mares

Donor mares should be examined on a routine basis to determine the optimal day to breed, confirm the day of ovulation, and schedule the day for the embryo flush procedure. Examinations are initiated on the second day of estrus or approximately 4 days after prostaglandin administration. Ultrasound examinations are subsequently performed daily once a developing follicle attains a diameter of approximately 30 mm. The donor mare can be bred when the dominant follicle is approximately 35 mm in diameter, depending on the breed. The ultimate goal is to inseminate the mare with fresh, cooled or frozen semen within 48, 24 or 12 hours prior to ovulation, respectively. If only a single dose of frozen semen is available, it may be preferred to inseminate immediately after ovulation is detected, which may require ultrasound examinations every 4 to 6 hours.

Human chorionic gonadotropin (**hCG**) or deslorelin acetate may be administered to mares in estrus to induce a timed ovulation. Administration of hCG (2,500 IU, i.v.) or deslorelin acetate (1.0 to 1.8 mg, i.m.) to a mare in estrus with a follicle ≥ 35 mm in diameter will generally induce ovulation in approximately 36 hours or 40 hours, respectively. The timing of administration of an ovulation inducing agent will often depend on the availability, type and quality of semen to be used.

Ultrasound examinations should continue to be performed daily to determine the day of ovulation and the number of ovulations, and to evaluate uterine health after insemination. Mares that accumulate fluid in their uterus after insemination should be treated (see below) to optimize embryo recovery.

Embryo collection should be scheduled based on the known ovulation date(s) and other factors, such as age of the donor mare, type of semen used, and information from previous embryo collection attempts. Embryo collection is usually performed on day 7 or day 8 after ovulation, although some clinicians prefer to flush a mare on day 9 and recover larger embryos. A flush on day 6.5 or early on day 7 may be preferred if the goal is to obtain a small embryo (i.e. < 300 µm) for cryopreservation. The collection attempt may be delayed for 12 to 24 hours for older mares (i.e. > 20 years of age) and mares bred with frozen semen.

Donor mares should be administered prostaglandins immediately after the flush procedure to lyse the corpus luteum and allow the mare to return to estrus. In addition, some veterinarians feel that it is important to examine the donor mare the day after the flush procedure to evaluate uterine health.

Reproductive Problems in Donor Mares

The most common reproductive problem encountered in embryo donor mares is accumulation of uterine fluid after insemination or persistent mating induced endometritis (**PMIE**). Other common problems include infectious endometritis and ovulation failure. A list of common and less common reproductive problems encountered in broodmare practice is presented in Table 4-1.

Table 4-1.
Common and less common reproductive problems of non-pregnant mares.

Common Reproductive Problems	Less Common Reproductive Problems
Behavior Adverse behavior when in estrus Silent heat	**Behavior** Persistent estrus Stallion-like behavior
Ovary Hemorrhagic anovulatory follicles Ovulation failure Persistent corpus luteum Premature luteolysis (endometritis)	**Ovary** Ovarian tumors Failure of follicular development
Oviduct Perovarian cysts	**Oviduct** Oviductal blockage Salpingitis
Uterus Persistent mating-induced endometritis Bacterial endometritis Uterine cysts Endometriosis	**Uterus** Fungal endometritis Pyometra Persistent endometrial cups Tumor (i.e. leiomyoma) Foreign body
Cervix Failure of cervical relaxation Cervical lacerations	**Cervix** Cervical adhesions Tumor (i.e. leiomyoma)
Vagina/Vestibule Urovagina Vericose veins Imperforate hymen	**Vagina/Vestibule** Lacerations Adhesions Vaginitis
Perineum Poor conformation Inadequate vulva tone Perineal lacerations Melanoma (grey mares)	**Perineum** Squamous cell carcinoma Coital exanthema (EHV-3)
Miscellaneous Cushing's disease	**Miscellaneous** Chromosomal abnormalities Mastitis Inappropriate lactation

Persistent uterine inflammation with fluid accumulation is common in individual middle aged to older mares (i.e. ≥ 15 years of age). The uterus will often appear normal on ultrasonographic evaluation prior to insemination and will contain a moderate to large volume of echogenic fluid the day after insemination. In most instances the inflammation is not due to a bacterial infection, but secondary to antigenic stimulation from spermatozoa. Treatment consists of uterine lavage using large volumes (1 to 3 liters) of sterile saline or lactated Ringer's solution **(LRS)** in conjunction with ecbolic agents such as oxytocin (10 to 20 units, IM or IV) or cloprostenol (250 µg, IM). Uterine lavage should continue until the effluent fluid is clear. Once a mare has exhibited clinical signs of PMIE, it is likely that the issue will reoccur following subsequent inseminations. Prevention of PMIE entails limiting the number of inseminations (i.e. preferably only one insemination), prophylactic uterine lavage 4 to 6 hours after insemination, and strategic administration of oxytocin or cloprostenol (see Formulary in Appendix).

Oxytocin causes uterine contractions for 30 to 45 minutes, while cloprostenol will cause uterine contractions for 2 to 4 hours. In some mares, either oxytocin or prostaglandins may work dramatically better than the other agent at elimination of uterine fluid. The choice of oxytocin or prostaglandins as an ecbolic agent often depends on the time of insemination, stage of cycle, previous efficacy in the mare to be treated, availability of assistance to administer additional doses, and clinician preference. Oxytocin or prostaglandins may be administered prior to ovulation without an adverse effect on development of the subsequent corpus luteum. In contract, administration of prostaglandins after ovulation will interfere with development of the corpus luteum and post-ovulation administration should therefore be avoided, if possible. If it is necessary to administer prostaglandins after ovulation to facilitate clearance of uterine fluid, the mare may be administered progesterone or altrenogest until the day of the embryo flush procedure. Dexamethasone (30 to 50 mg, IV) may also be administered at the time of insemination to reduce the uterine inflammatory response to spermatozoal challenge.

Infectious endometritis is most commonly due to bacterial organisms and less commonly due to fungal organisms. The most common bacterial organisms associated with equine endometritis include *Streptococcus equi* subspecies *zooepidemicus*, *Escherichia coli*, *Klebsiella pneumoniae* and *Pseudomonas aeruginosa*. The most common fungal organisms are *Candida albicans* and *Aspergillus fumigatus*. A clinical suspicion or diagnosis of infectious endometritis may be made by a combination of ultrasonography (presence of echogenic fluid in the uterus), presence of inflammatory cells (i.e. neutrophils) on uterine cytology, growth of organism(s) on culture, and detection of bacterial or fungal DNA on polymerase chain reaction **(PCR)** analysis of a uterine sample. Treatment may consist of uterine lavage to remove debris, fluid and organisms, infusion of antimicrobial agents into the uterine lumen for 3 to 5 days, and possibly systemic administration of antimicrobial agents. Selection of an antimicrobial agent should be based on *in vitro* susceptibility tests. Dosage and routes of administration of common antibiotic and antifungal agents is presented in the Formulary (see Appendix). Prevention of infectious endometritis is based on correction of predisposing factors, such as a Caslick procedure in mares with poor perineal conformation or inadequate vulvar tone. Strict adherence to principles of hygiene, use of sterile equipment, and evaluation of the mare after insemination and embryo collection procedures will serve to minimize uterine contamination and infection.

Additional Donor Management Considerations

It is recommended that a donor mare be allowed to carry a foal to term at least once by the time she is 8 to 10 years of age. In addition, it is recommended that a donor mare be allowed to carry her own foal to term every 3 to 4 years. The ultimate goal is to optimize the reproductive health of the donor mare over her lifetime. A mare can be an embryo donor prior to and after carrying and giving birth to her own foal.

Mares that are never allowed to carry their own foal may eventually develop issues with abnormal cervical function, leading to chronic accumulation of inflammatory fluid in their uterus. This is noted in older maiden mares as well as middle-aged to older mares used solely as embryo donors. Anecdotal clinical evidence suggests that normal cervical function is maintained in donor mares allowed to occasionally carry their own foal to term.

Clinical research has provided evidence that repeated cycles of insemination and embryo collection may predispose donor mares to uterine inflammation and infection. Individual mares may be adversely affected by the third to fifth cycle of insemination and embryo collection. Affected mares tend to accumulate a small to moderate volume of echogenic fluid in their uterus, have inflammatory cells present on uterine cytology, and yield a light to moderate growth of one or more bacterial organisms on uterine culture.

As a consequence, close attention should be paid to the uterine health of individual donor mares in an embryo transfer program. Uterine culture and cytology samples should be collected and evaluated from donor mares with any accumulation of fluid in their uterine lumen. Early treatment should be instituted on mares with confirmed uterine infections and occasionally a mare may require a cycle off to allow for uterine treatment.

Older maiden mares and early post-partum mares offer challenges in an embryo transfer program. An older maiden mare may have a cervix that fails to relax during estrus. This may lead to accumulation of a significant volume of inflammatory fluid following insemination and hence a poor uterine environment for survival of an embryo. Anticipation of cervical issues is the key to successful reproductive management of an older maiden mare. A vaginal speculum examination and a digital (manual) examination of the cervix when the mare is in heat will determine the degree of cervical relaxation and the probability of uterine fluid accumulation after breeding. Mares at risk should be bred or inseminated only once, preferably just prior to ovulation. A timed ovulation can be induced by administration of hCG or deslorelin when a follicle of the optimal size is present during mid-estrus. The uterus should be lavaged 4 to 6 hours after breeding to remove residual sperm, inflammatory cells and fluid from the uterine lumen. Administration of one or more doses of oxytocin may also be helpful to promote uterine contractions and evacuation of uterine fluid.

Pregnancy and embryo recovery rates may be acceptable for mares bred on their first post-partum estrus (foal heat) if parturition was uneventful, fetal membranes were not retained, there was no prolonged period of lochial discharge, and ovulation did not occur prior to day 10 postpartum. Embryo collection can be successful early in the post-partum period, but the flush procedure is often associated with a large amount of uterine debris. It may be better to allow the mare to go through her foal heat, administer prostaglandins approximately 5 days after ovulation and breed the mare for embryo collection on the subsequent estrus or wait until the second post-partum estrus (30-day heat).

Recommended Reading

LeBlanc MM. When to refer an infertile mare to a theriogenologist. Theriogenology 2008; 70: 421-429.

McCue PM. The problem mare: management philosophy, diagnostic procedures, and therapeutic options. J Eq Vet Sci 2008; 28:619-626.

Pycock JF. Breeding management of the problem mare. In: Equine Breeding Management and Artificial Insemination, Samper JC, Ed. WB Saunders, Philadelphia, 2000, pp 195-228.

Squires EL, Seidel Jr., GE Collection and transfer of equine embryos. Colorado State University Animal Reproduction and Biotechnology Laboratory Bulletin No. 8, 1995; 64 pp.

CHAPTER 5

SUPEROVULATION

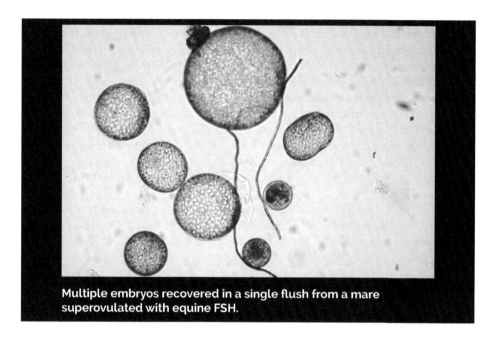

Multiple embryos recovered in a single flush from a mare superovulated with equine FSH.

Introduction

Embryos are recovered from donor mares with single ovulations on approximately 50 to 65% of cycles. Presuming that the fertility potential of the mare and stallion are not at issue, the only way to significantly improve embryo recovery is to stimulate development and ovulation of multiple follicles. A goal in the horse breeding industry has been to develop a protocol to increase ovulation rate without adversely affecting embryo collection rate per ovulation.

A Brief History of Superovulation in the Mare

Attempts at inducing ovulation of multiple follicles have included administration of equine chorionic gonadotropin **(ecG)**, gonadotropin releasing hormone **(GnRH)** or GnRH agonists, porcine follicle stimulating hormone **(pFSH)**, equine pituitary extract **(EPE)**, purified equine FSH **(eFSH)** and recombinant equine FSH **(reFSH)**. In addition, mares have been actively immunized against inhibin or administered inhibin antiserum in an attempt to induce multiple ovulations. Administration of ecG, GnRH and pFSH are not effective in consistent stimulation of follicular development in the cycling mare. Administration of GnRH or pFSH twice daily has been reported to increase the percentage of mares with double-ovulations. Active or passive immunization against inhibin is not practical or commercially available at this time.

The only successful and repeatable treatment protocol for superovulation of mares has been administration of eFSH (Bioniche Animal Health, Bogart, Georgia) or reFSH (AspenBio Pharma Inc., Castle Rock, Colorado). Unfortunately, at the present time, neither product is commercially available or approved for use in the horse.

Recombinant Equine FSH

A recombinant equine FSH (reFSH) preparation has been developed which is comprised of a single chain chimera with the amino terminus of the equine FSH alpha subunit and the carboxyl end of the equine FSH beta subunit attached to each other using the carboxyl terminal peptide of eCG/eLH beta. reFSH has been shown to have biological activity both *in vitro* and *in vivo*.

Potential advantages of a recombinant preparation include purity, sterility and consistency of FSH bioactivity. Research studies have demonstrated that reFSH can initiate follicular development in seasonally anestrous mares and stimulate development of multiple follicles in cycling mares (Figure 5-1). An average of 2.5 to 4.0 ovulations per cycle has been reported using reFSH in cycling mares.

However, not every mare treated with reFSH has ovulated multiple follicles or donated embryo(s). The variability in response has been attributed to one or more of the following factors:
1. Individual response of mare
2. Individual endogenous FSH levels
3. Inappropriate timing of FSH treatments
4. Age of mare
5. Fertility of semen used for insemination

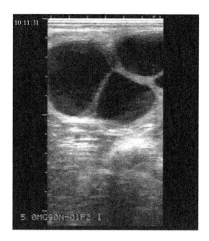

Figure 5-1. Ultrasound image of an ovary with multiple large follicles in a mare treated with reFSH.

6. Depression in endogenous LH as a result of high estradiol and inhibin levels
7. Failure of oocytes to mature

Protocol for Superovulation with eFSH or reFSH

The most consistent and productive strategy has been to initiate exogenous FSH therapy when a cohort of follicles in a follicular wave is beginning to develop and endogenous FSH is beginning to decline. The goal is to "rescue" the subordinate follicles that would otherwise undergo atresia after follicle deviation.

The protocol for stimulation of development of multiple follicles in cycling mares is as follows:
• Examine mares with ultrasound once daily beginning 5 days after ovulation
• Allow endogenous FSH to initiate follicular development
• Start FSH therapy when one or more follicles first reach 15 to 20 mm in diameter, continue therapy every 12 hours
• Administer prostaglandins (i.e. cloprostenol) on day 2 of FSH treatment
• Continue administration of FSH every 12 h until the majority of follicles are 30 to 35 mm in diameter, then discontinue FSH treatments
• Allow a "coast period" of 30 to 36 hours during which no treatments are administered
• Administer hCG to induce synchronized ovulation of follicle(s)

Factors Affecting Response to FSH

Size of Follicles. The main factor determining the response to FSH is the number and size of follicles present on the ovary at the initiation of FSH treatment. A long duration of FSH therapy can be expected if all follicles are < 10 mm in diameter at onset of treatment. Consequently it may be more cost effective to allow endogenous FSH to stimulate initial follicular development. The highest ovulation rate has been shown to be in mares with a large number of follicles 15 to 20 mm at the time treatment is initiated. Mares with a follicle ≥ 25 mm at onset of treatment usually only have one ovulation. Consequently, it is a waste of FSH and money to treat a mare that has already gone through follicular deviation, so an ultrasound examination should always be performed prior to a decision to initiate treatment. FSH therapy should be discontinued once follicle(s) are ≥ 35 mm in diameter. Additional FSH therapy may not be cost effective and may be associated with a higher rate of ovulation failure.

Treatment Frequency
Administration of FSH twice per day results in higher ovulation rates than once per day treatment.

Follicle Coasting
The "coast period" is the interval between FSH treatment and administration of an ovulation induction agent. The intent of the coast period is to prevent overstimulation of follicles, decrease the incidence of ovulation failure, and minimize the number of doses of FSH required.

Potential Problems Associated with FSH Treatment
• Failure of all dominant follicles to ovulate in response to hCG
• Formation of anovulatory follicles
• Development and ovulation of only one follicle
• Poor embryo recovery despite a good ovulation response

Suggested Reading
Squires EL and McCue PM. 2011. Superovulation. In: McKinnon AO, Squires EL, Vaala WE, and Varner DD (Eds). Equine Reproduction, Second Edition; Wiley-Blackwell, Ames, Iowa; 2011: Pp. 1836-1845.

Meyers-Brown G, McCue PM, Niswender KD, Squires EL, DeLuca CA, Bidstrup LA, Colgin M, Famula TR and Roser JF. Superovulation in mares using recombinant equine follicle stimulating hormones: ovulation rates, embryo retrieval and hormone profiles. J Equine Vet Sci. 2010; 30:560-568.

Welsh SA, Denniston DJ, Hudson JJ, Bruemmer JE, McCue PM, Squires EL. Exogenous eFSH, follicle coasting, and hCG as a novel superovulation regimen in mares. J Equine Vet Sci . 2006; 26:262-270.

CHAPTER 6

EMBRYO COLLECTION

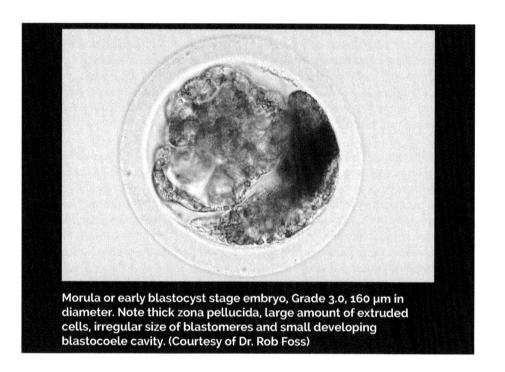

Morula or early blastocyst stage embryo, Grade 3.0, 160 µm in diameter. Note thick zona pellucida, large amount of extruded cells, irregular size of blastomeres and small developing blastocoele cavity. (Courtesy of Dr. Rob Foss)

Introduction

Embryo recovery attempts may be successfully performed 6.5 to 9 days after ovulation. A collection attempt may be performed on day 6 or early on day 7 to procure small (i.e. < 300 μm) embryos for cryopreservation. A majority of mares are flushed on day 7 or 8 post ovulation because embryo recovery rates are high and a majority of embryos are expanded blastocysts and are therefore easily observed under the microscope. The collection procedure is often delayed by one-half day for older mares and mares bred with frozen semen because of the perception of a slight delay in embryonic development. For example, a morula-stage embryo may be recovered from a mare bred with frozen semen on day 8 after ovulation when one would normally expect a blastocyst or expanded blastocyst stage embryo. It is possible that the embryo may not have been in the uterus if the mare had been flushed on the morning of day 7. Embryo collection attempts on day 9 after ovulation may result in the recovery of large embryos (i.e. > 1 to 2 mm in diameter) that are easily damaged during handling and transfer. Equipment and supplies needed for embryo collection are presented in Table 6-1.

The mare is typically restrained in examination stocks during the embryo collection procedure. However, in some instances a mare may be flushed in a stall or other area provided that appropriate safety precautions are considered. A majority of donor mares do not require sedation to safely and effectively perform the uterine flush procedure. Sedation may be warranted in young, small, excited or dangerous mares. Options for sedation include acepromazine, xylazine hydrochloride and detomidine hydrochloride. A combination of xylazine or detomidine plus butorphanol tartrate may be beneficial in some mares.

Table 6-1
Equipment and Supplies

Recommended Equipment and Supplies:	Additional Equipment and Supplies:
Catheter	Sedation
Y-tubing or other tubing	Buscopan®
Embryo filter	Oxytocin
Embryo flush media	Ultrasound unit
Graduated cylinder	
Syringe (60 mls)	

A sterile catheter, typically 80 cm in length and 8.0 mm internal diameter, with an inflatable cuff is used for the lavage (Figure 6-1). Sterile "Y-tubing", with clamps to regulate inflow and outflow, is used to connect the uterine catheter to a container of flush media and to an embryo filter (Figure 6-2). Several types of embryo filters, each with a 75 μm screen, are commercially available (Figure 6-3A, B, C and D). Options include filters with a mesh screen on the bottom, on the side, or on a raised area in the center. Some filters also function as a search dish, while others require that the contents be poured into a separate search dish.

Historically, many facilities made their own embryo flush media from bulk chemicals and added antibiotics to control bacterial growth. Either fetal or newborn calf serum

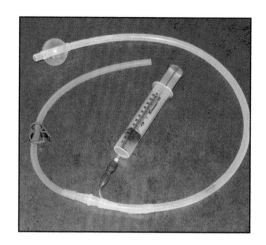

Figure 6-1. Uterine lavage catheter with cuff inflated with air.

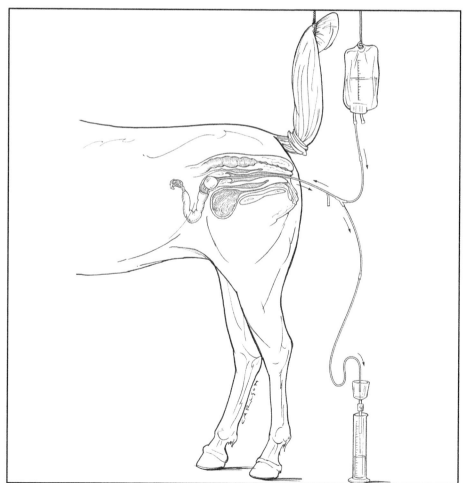

Figure 6-2. Non-surgical embryo collection procedure. Note that the cuff of the uterine catheter is inflated and positioned against the internal os of the cervix. Y-tubing connects the catheter to a vessel of flush media and the embryo filter.

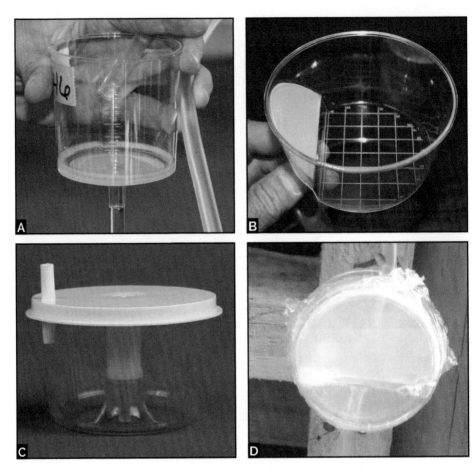

Figure 6-3. A. Embryo filter with screen on the bottom. **B.** Embryo filter with screen on the side. **C.** Embryo filter with screen in the center. **D.** Embryo filter with screen in center.

was added as a surfactant to prevent the embryo from adhering to the catheter, filter or search dish. This was followed by the use of commercially prepared Dulbecco's phosphate buffered saline (PBS) to which antibiotics and either fresh or lyophilized calf serum was added. The equine ET industry in the United States has now largely shifted to the use of commercially prepared "complete" flush media (non-PBS) that contains a Zwitterion-based buffer system, antibiotics and purified albumen or polyvinyl alcohol (PVA) as a surfactant (Figure 6-4). Lactated Ringer's solution (LRS) or equivalent may also be used as an embryo flush medium with or without the addition of either calf serum or bovine serum albumen (BSA) as a surfactant. LRS-type fluids have been used in Argentina and Brazil for many years with good embryo collection rates and good pregnancy rates following transfer, but there have been no studies published to directly compare LRS with commercial embryo flush media.

Embryo Collection Procedure

The uterine flush technique and equipment are often dictated by the preferences of the clinician or technician. The procedure must be performed in a clean and safe environment.

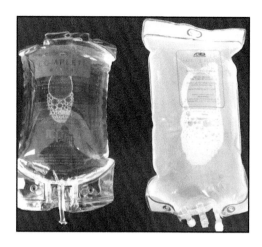

Figure 6-4. Examples of complete embryo flush media.

The tail is wrapped and manure in the rectum is removed to facilitate uterine massage that is often performed per rectum during the flush procedure. The perineum of the mare is washed a minimum of three times with a non-residual soap, rinsed thoroughly with fresh water and dried with paper towels. The vestibule should also be swabbed with a pledget of moist cotton or paper towels to remove organic debris that may contaminate the mare or flush medium.

Donor mares with a history of infectious endometritis or retention of uterine fluid after insemination should be examined by ultrasound prior to the flush attempt to confirm the presence or absence of uterine fluid. If a significant volume of echogenic fluid is present, the embryo flush procedure should be cancelled as the likelihood of obtaining a viable embryo is extremely low.

The standard method of embryo collection in the mare is a nonsurgical, transcervical uterine lavage. The catheter is gently inserted through the cervix, which should be tightly closed in a diestrous mare, and into the caudal uterine body. The cuff is subsequently inflated with 60 to 75 mls of air using a syringe. The catheter is then gently pulled caudally to "lock" the cuff against the internal cervical os. If the cuff is not inflated properly the catheter may not remain in the uterus. Similarly, if the cuff is inflated within the cervical lumen, the catheter may be expelled from the reproductive tract when flush media is infused. If the catheter is extended too far into the uterus, the cuff may be inflated within one horn and only that horn would be lavaged.

There are many techniques utilized to successfully remove an embryo. A common technique is to lavage the uterus of a donor mare three times sequentially with a total of 3 to 4 liters of media, using up to 1 to 2 liters each time. The media may be prewarmed (i.e. 30-37° C) or used at room temperature. The amount of fluid used for each flush is dependent on the size of the uterus, parity of the mare and preference of the clinician. Young maiden mares may only be able to hold 400 to 500 mls before becoming uncomfortable or inflow ceases. In contrast, mares that have had a foal previously may easily hold 1 to 2 liters of media. The goal is to expand the uterine lumen sufficiently to allow fluid to effectively reach all parts of the uterus, including the area between endometrial folds. The donor mare may become mildly uncomfortable upon stretching of the perimetrium and this can be used to indicate that sufficient infusion of fluid into the uterus has occurred. The flush medium is then allowed to egress back out the catheter by gravity flow through the embryo filter. An alternative is to collect the effluent fluid in the original vessel and then pour the contents through an embryo filter.

The embryo filter cup may be directly connected to the effluent portion of "Y" tubing creating a "closed" system (Figure 6-5). Alternatively, the top of the filter cup may be discarded and the effluent tubing manually held within the cup in an "open" system (Figure 6-6). With an open system, care must be taken to not overflow the cup.

The uterus of the mare is often massaged per rectum during infusion and recovery of the media to ensure that fluid fills each uterine horn. Some clinicians massage the uterus during each round of lavages while others only massage the uterus during recovery of the final liter of media. Administration of a medication (i.e. Buscopan®) to relax the rectal musculature and relieve straining may help facilitate the massage procedure.

Recovery of uterine lavage fluid may be monitored by collection of effluent into graduated cylinders (Figure 6-7). The volume of fluid infused into the uterus can be

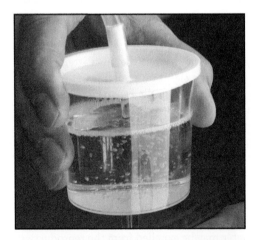

Figure 6-5. "Closed" system of embryo collection with "Y" tubing attached to filter cap.

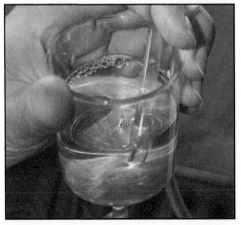

Figure 6-6. "Open" system of embryo collection with "Y" tubing not directly attached to filter.

compared to the amount of fluid recovered to determine if a significant volume of fluid is still present in the uterus. Alternatively, the uterus may be examined by transrectal ultrasonography at the conclusion of the flush procedure to confirm that all of the media has been evacuated. Oxytocin (20 IU, intravenously) may be administered during the flush procedure to stimulate uterine contractions and aid in fluid recovery.

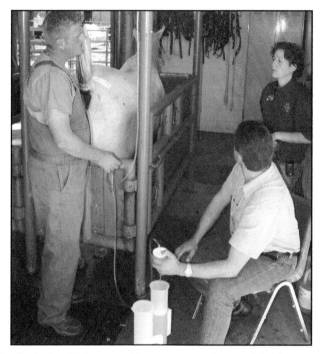

Figure 6-7. Graduated cylinders used to measure volume of fluid recovered during an embryo collection procedure.

An alternative embryo collection technique is to infuse 500 to 1,000 mls of flush media into the uterus through a single tube connecting the media container (i.e. bag or bottle) with the uterine catheter. This is accomplished by simply raising the media container above the level of the uterus (Figure 6-8). The container is then lowered below the level of the uterus and fluid is recovered into the original container by gravity flow (Figure 6-9). This is repeated for a total of three infusions, after which the fluid recovered into the 3 individual containers is poured through a filter (Figure 6-10) and examined under a microscope.

Problems Associated with the Flush Attempt

The primary problem encountered during the embryo collection attempt is interruption of fluid outflow due to endometrial tissue or endometrial cysts obstructing the catheter. Gentle rotation (180° to 360°), advancement and other movements of the catheter may be sufficient to free the endometrium from the catheter.

Another common issue is failure to retrieve all of the medium infused into the uterus. Ultrasound examination will reveal the volume and location of the medium within

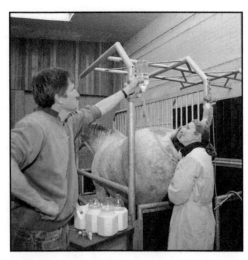

Figure 6-8. Bottle flush technique. A one liter bottle of flush media is raised and the media is allowed to enter the uterus by gravity flow. (Photo courtesy of Dr. Peter Daels)

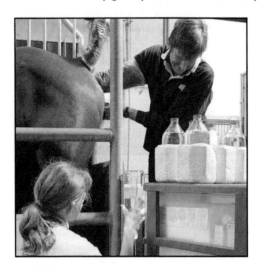

Figure 6-9. Lowering the bottle to recover media and embryo from the uterus. (Photo courtesy of Dr. Peter Daels)

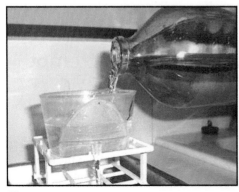

Figure 6-10. Pouring contents of the media bottle through an embryo filter. (Photo courtesy of Dr. Peter Daels)

the uterine lumen. A technique to retrieve the fluid includes deflation of the cuff, advancement of the catheter into the fluid pocket, massage of the uterus per rectum or adding more fluid to the uterus to "restart" the siphon effect. Fluid recovery can be monitored by transrectal ultrasound during the collection process (Figure 6-11).

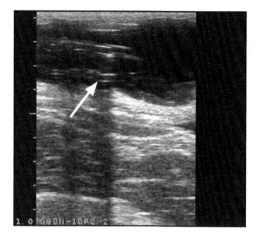

Figure 6-11. Ultrasound photo of embryo fluid collection. Note the dual set of parallel echogenic lines (arrow) indicating the presence of the silastic catheter entering the fluid filled uterus from the left.

Searching for an Embryo

Search for an embryo may occur after each successive lavage or after the final volume of media is recovered. Occasionally a large expanded blastocyst-stage embryo may be directly visualized in the filter cup. However, in most instances the embryo is identified with the aid of a stereo microscope. The quality of microscope is a key factor in the success of an embryo transfer program. Ideally the microscope should have the following characteristics:
• Quality optics
• Variable zoom capability (10x to 50x)
• Base illumination without heat production
• Mirror (for oblique illumination and contrast enhancement)
• Linear metric eyepiece micrometer; calibrated at common points of magnification
• Large enough base surface to accommodate search dishes and embryo manipulation

The contents of the filter are poured into a round sterile disposable plastic search dish approximately 60 mm in diameter (Figure 6-12). Some embryo filters are designed to also serve as the search dish. The outflow port is occluded with a plug (provided) to allow the filter/dish to be placed onto the stage glass of the microscope without leakage of fluid (Figure 6-13). Search dishes should have a grid on the bottom to allow for a systematic search for the embryo. Petri dishes can be purchased with a grid already present on the bottom (Figure 6-14) or a grid can be placed on the bottom using a scalpel blade (Figure 6-15).

The filter is then rinsed with 20 to 30 mls of flush medium saved for this purpose (Figure 6-16). A gentle swirling motion of a round search dish may be used to move the embryo and cellular debris to the center of the search dish (Figure 6-17). The embryo and cellular debris will gradually sink to the bottom of the dish, so the focus of the microscope should be directed in that plane.

The dish is then examined for the presence of an embryo, unfertilized oocyte, amount of cellular debris, etc. The search often begins in the center of the dish, as the swirling usually moves the embryo to that location, if properly performed.

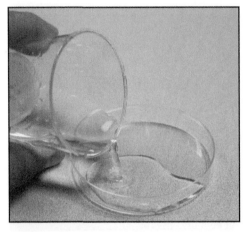

Figure 6-12. Contents of an embryo filter being poured into a search dish.

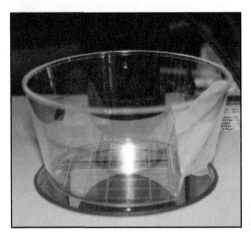

Figure 6-13. Embryo filter that is also a search dish.

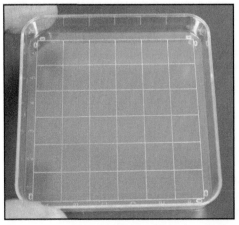

Figure 6-14. A square embryo search dish with grid on bottom.

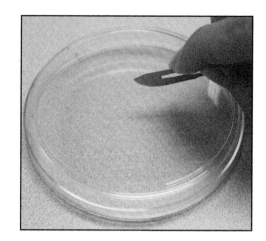

Figure 6-15. Creating a grid on the bottom of a round plastic petri dish using a scalpel blade.

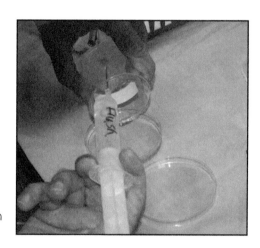

Figure 6-16. Rinsing the filter with flush medium.

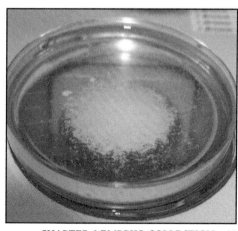

Figure 6-17. Swirling the search dish moved cellular debris and hopefully the embryo into the center.

If an embryo is not immediately located, the entire dish should be systematically searched using the grid lines for orientation. Debris may be moved out of the way using a sterile needle or other small sterile device (Figure 6-18).

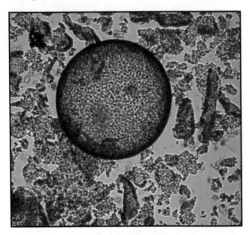

Figure 6-18. Embryo located amidst cellular debris.

Embryo Collection Rate

In a retrospective analysis of 492 embryo collection procedures performed on client mares, the average number of ovulations per cycle and number of embryos recovered per flush were 1.18 ± 0.02 and 0.52 ± 0.03, respectively. Embryo recovery rates per flush and per ovulation were 48.1% and 45.2%, respectively.

A majority of embryos (97.6 %) recovered were of excellent (Grade 1) or good (Grade 2) quality (Table 6-2). Average size (outer diameter) of the embryo approximately doubled with each successive collection day (Table 6-3). Percentages of embryos in various developmental stages (morula, early blastocyst, blastocyst, and expanded blastocyst) are presented in Table 6-4.

Table 6-2.
Embryo quality score (grade) for embryos collected from donor mares.

Grade	Comment	# Embryos	Percentage (%)
1	Excellent	198	78.9%
2	Good	47	18.7%
3	Poor	6	2.4%
4	Degenerate or Dead	0	0%

Table 6-3.
Diameter (µm) of embryos relative to day of the collection procedure.

Collection Day	# Embryos	Mean ± S.D. (µm)	Range (µm)
6	20	191.8 ± 13.2	150-325
7	183	354.0 ± 13.9	150-900
8	35	623.9 ± 72.9	150-2,500

Table 6-4.
Stage and size of embryonic development for embryos collected from donor mares on the afternoon of day 7.

Stage	# Embryos	Percentage (%)	Mean ± S.D. (μm)	Range (μm)
Morula	31	12.2	156.7 ± 3.0	125-200
Early Blastocyst	66	25.9	188.5 ± 3.9	150-225
Blastocyst	44	17.3	295.9 ± 6.3	200-400
Expanded blastocyst	115	45.1	598.0 ± 22.5	250-2,500

Re-Flush Options

Unfortunately, a standard uterine lavage procedure is not always successful in recovering the embryo from an early pregnant mare. The possibility that an embryo may still be present in the uterus after an embryo collection attempt is not new. Several published reports have noted pregnancies that were established in mares from which no embryos were recovered during an embryo collection procedure. Other studies have reported that additional flushes per collection attempt increased the probability of recovering an embryo. Embryos were recovered from 9.5% of mares from which no embryos were recovered during an initial flush attempt following uterine lavage with an additional 3 liters of media. In addition, extra embryos were collected from superovulated mares following uterine lavage with an additional 3 liters of media (6 liters total).

Same Day Re-Flush

Consequently, if an embryo is not recovered following the initial series of lavages, 1 to 2 additional liters of media may be immediately infused into the uterus and 20 units of oxytocin is administered intravenously. The media is allowed to remain in the mare for approximately 3 minutes before being allowed to exit by gravity flow aided by uterine massage per rectum. The media is passed through an embryo filter, the content of which is subsequently examined under a microscope. This procedure will increase overall embryo recovery rate by 5 to 15%. The increased embryo recovery rate provided by a "same day re-flush" is economically significant in a clinical embryo transfer program. The cost of the additional media, oxytocin and clinician time is usually minimal compared with the potential value of a recovered embryo. In addition, mares are typically only managed through 3 to 5 estrous cycles per year. Each cycle is important and embryo recovery rates should be optimized on each cycle. In addition, it is not possible to predict with absolute certainty, if another good opportunity to collect an embryo will be available that season.

Next Day Re-Flush

Limited published data are available to evaluate the efficacy of re-flushing an individual mare the day after the original flush procedure. Next day re-flushes are not routinely performed or recommended in clinical practice. Situations in which the procedure may be indicated are the last cycle of the year, if an unfertilized oocyte was recovered the previous day without concomitant recovery of an embryo, or in superovulated mares in which the rate of embryo recovery is less than 50% of the number of ovulations detected. A retrospective study evaluated the embryo recovery rate for next day re-flushes on 31 mares with negative flushes the previous day. A total of 2 liters of media were infused into the uterus, 20 IU of oxytocin was administered intravenously and the fluid was allowed to remain in the uterus for 3 minutes. Embryos were recovered on 3 of the 31 flushes (9.7%). In general, the recovered fluid was slightly cloudy and mild to moderate debris was present in the search dish.

Prostaglandin Administration after Embryo Collection Procedure

It is recommended that prostaglandins (i.e. cloprostenol sodium, 250 µg, IM) be administered after each embryo collection procedure. The goal is to lyse the corpus luteum and allow the mare to come back into estrus. This will facilitate evacuation of any fluid remaining in the uterus and minimize the adverse consequences of inadvertently introducing bacteria into the uterus of a diestrous mare. Administration of prostaglandins will also shorten the luteal phase and thereby allow an earlier opportunity to rebreed the mare if another ET cycle is warranted. In addition, short-cycling will minimize or eliminate the possibility that a pregnancy will continue in the donor mare if the embryo collection attempt was negative. An exception to this guideline is if an owner decides to allow the mare to carry the pregnancy in the event that an embryo was not recovered during a flush procedure (Figure 6-19).

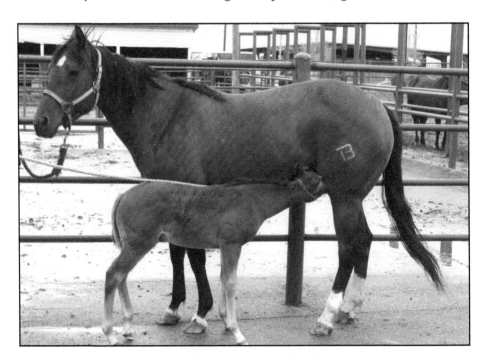

Figure 6-19. Foal born 330 days after a negative embryo collection attempt. The owner elected to not administer prostaglandins after the flush attempt. An ultrasound examination 7 days later revealed that the mare was pregnant.

Recommended Reading

McCue PM, Niswender KD, Macon KA. Modification of the flush procedure to enhance embryo recovery. J Equine Vet Sci 2003; 23:1-2.

Squires EL, Seidel Jr., GE. Collection and transfer of equine embryos. Colorado State University Animal Reproduction and Biotechnology Laboratory Bulletin No. 8, 1995; 64 pp.

CHAPTER 7

FACTORS AFFECTING
EMBRYO RECOVERY

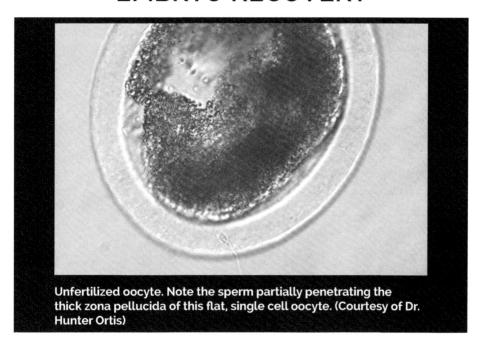

Unfertilized oocyte. Note the sperm partially penetrating the thick zona pellucida of this flat, single cell oocyte. (Courtesy of Dr. Hunter Ortis)

Introduction

Embryo recovery rate is influenced by many factors including reproductive health and age of the donor mare, semen type and quality, flush technique, number of flushes performed during the season, day of embryo recovery attempt, number of ovulations and clinical expertise.

Reproductive Health of the Donor Mare

On average, equine embryos are recovered from approximately 50 to 65% of collection attempts. Embryo collection success may approach 70 to 75% per cycle from young reproductively healthy donor mares bred with good quality semen. In contrast, embryo recovery may average 20 to 30% per cycle in mares with a history of reproductive problems.

Persistent mating-induced endometritis **(PMIE)** has an adverse effect on embryo recovery. In a retrospective study, donor mares with limited to no fluid in their uterus 24 hours after breeding yielded an embryo on 158 of 307 flushes (51.5%), while embryos were recovered on 78 of 176 cycles (44.3%) in which mild to moderate echogenic fluid was present after breeding (p=0.1016). Mares in the latter category were typically managed by a combination of uterine lavage and ecbolic agents (i.e. oxytocin or prostaglandins) (Figure 7-1).

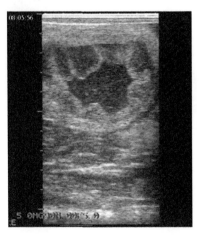

Figure 7-1. Ultrasound photograph of an embryo donor mare with persistent mating induced endometritis. Note the large volume of echogenic fluid within the uterine lumen.

Similarly, the quality or character of the embryo flush media recovered during a collection attempt is associated with embryo recovery success (Figure 7-2). Mares with minimal debris in the uterine effluent yielded an embryo on 235 of 462 flushes (50.9%), while embryos were only recovered from 2 of 21 flushes (9.5%) when the media recovered was cloudy or contained an abnormally large amount of debris (p < 0.001).

Age of the Donor Mare

In another retrospective study, embryo recovery rate per flush from donor mares ≤ 15 years of age was 57.1% (144 of 252 flushes). In contrast, embryo recovery rate per flush was only 39.4% (93 of 236) from donor mares > 15 years of age. Reasons for the

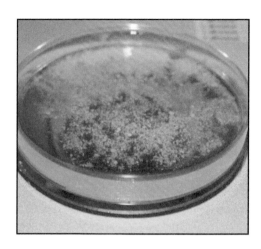

Figure 7-2. Large amount of debris within the search dish of a mare with persistent mating induced endometritis.

lower embryo recovery from old mares could be poor oocyte quality, a lower rate of fertilization, embryonic loss within the oviduct or embryonic loss within the uterus, or a poor uterine environment.

Oocytes from older mares have been noted to be of lower quality than oocytes from younger mares and oocyte quality may contribute to the high rate of early embryonic loss and lower embryo recovery rate (Figure 7-3).

Fertilization rates have been reported to be similar between old mares and young mares based on recovery of early cleavage-stage embryos from the oviduct 2 days after ovulation. However, embryo recovery from the uterus at 14 days of gestation was significantly lower in aged mares (20%) as compared to young mares (80%). This suggests that early embryonic loss is a major factor in older mares.

Oviductal abnormalities of mares are difficult to assess. Oviductal problems that may be associated with increased age and may be associated with decreased fertilization or increased embryonic loss include salpingitis and blockage. Techniques for evaluating oviductal problems include laparoscopy, application of starch granules or fluorescent

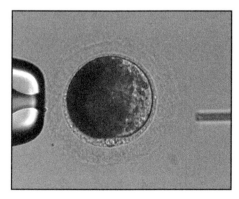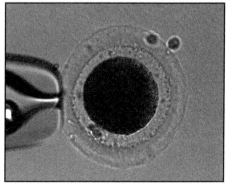

Figure 7-3. Oocytes collected via transvaginal aspiration from the ovary of a young mare (left) and an aged mare (right). (Oocyte photographs courtesy of Dr. Elaine Carnevale and JoAnne Stokes, Colorado State University).

microbeads to the infundibulum and monitoring oviductal passage into the uterus, flushing the oviductal lumen, and application of PGE_2 gel to the external surface of the oviduct.

Aged mares may exhibit a variety of uterine abnormalities that may be associated with decreased embryo survival, including persistent mating-induced endometritis, bacterial endometritis, fungal endometritis, endometrosis, and endometrial cysts. Fortunately, a majority of uterine issues can be diagnosed using a combination of ultrasonography, culture, cytology and biopsy.

Semen Type

Semen type can influence both the embryo recovery rate and the diameter of an embryo collected on a given flush day. Embryo recovery rates for mares inseminated with fresh or cooled-transported semen are typically higher than rates for mares bred with frozen semen. For example, mares inseminated with fresh or cooled-transported semen yielded one or more embryos on 51.9% (27/52) and 51.6% (182/353) of cycles, respectively, in a retrospective study. In contrast, mares bred with frozen semen donated one or more embryos on 33.3% of cycles (26/78).

Insemination of mares with frozen semen is also associated with recovery of smaller embryos on a given collection day as compared with insemination with fresh or cooled-transported semen. For example, diameter of embryos recovered on day 7 (n = 114) from mares bred with cooled semen (401.9 ± 19.6 μm) was larger ($p < 0.05$) than embryos recovered on day 7 from mares (n = 11) bred with frozen semen (258.2 ± 33.3 μm) (Figure 7-4). Similarly, embryos (n=24) collected on day 8 from mares bred with cooled semen tended ($p = 0.0553$) to be larger (716.9 ± 104.9 μm) than embryos (n = 10) collected on day 8 from mares bred with frozen semen (383.5 ± 54.9 μm). As a consequence, practitioners may opt to perform an embryo collection attempt on day 8 or 9 in mares bred with frozen semen in order to optimize recovery success. It is hypothesized that the difference in embryo diameter may be due to a delay in fertilization or a delay in early embryonic development associated with the use of frozen semen.

Embryo Collection Day

A majority of embryo recovery attempts are performed on day 7 or day 8 after ovulation. The reasons for flushing on day 7 or 8 include:
• Equine embryos do not enter the uterus until day 5.5 or 6
• Embryo recovery rate on day 6 is lower than on day 7 or later
• Embryos recovered on day 9 are often quite large and may be damaged during recovery, handling, washing, or transfer

Embryo recovery rate is similar for flush attempts performed on day 7 or 8. In contrast, the recovery rate is approximately 10 to 15% lower for attempts performed on day 6 after ovulation. The lower recovery rate for day 6 embryos may be due to inefficiency of the flush procedure to recover a small embryo, failure of some embryos to have entered the uterus from the oviduct by day 6, or failure to identify a small embryo in the search dish.

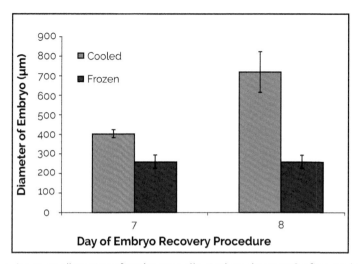

Figure 7-4. Average diameter of embryos collected on day 7 or 8 after ovulation from mares inseminated with cooled-transported semen or frozen semen.

The primary reason for performing an embryo flush procedure 6 days after ovulation is to collect a small embryo for cryopreservation. Equine embryos begin to expand on day 7 and approximately double in size between days 7 and 8 after ovulation and double again in diameter between days 8 and 9. Some clinicians prefer to flush mares on day 8 or 9 with the intent of collecting a large expanded blastocyst. A delay in embryonic development may occur in some older mares and in mares bred with frozen semen. It may be beneficial to flush those mares on day 8 or 9 to optimize recovery.

Flush Technique

It is common for a clinician to have a standardized embryo collection technique. However, the technique should be adjusted according to specific circumstances for individual donor mares.

For example, it is possible to infuse 1 to 2 liters of media into the uterus of barren, open and foaling mares. In contrast, a young maiden mare may only allow 400 to 500 mls of fluid into her uterus before she becomes uncomfortable and anxious. A common practice is to infuse and recover approximately 1 liter of media into the uterus of the donor mare on 3 successive procedures before searching for the embryo. It was reported in one study that 57.1% of embryos collected were recovered after infusion and recovery of the first liter, 23.8% of embryos were recovered after the second liter and 19.0% were detected after the third liter of fluid.

Subsequently, if no embryo is recovered after the first round of uterine lavages, and the estrous cycle of the donor mare was judged to be good and the semen quality was adequate, it may be beneficial to flush the mare again. Clinical trials have demonstrated that embryo recovery can be enhanced by 5 to 15% by immediately performing an additional flush procedure. Media is infused into the uterus of the donor mare, she is administered 20 units of oxytocin intravenously, and the fluid is allowed to remain in the uterus for 3 minutes. The uterus is massaged per rectum to facilitate fluid recovery.

The reason(s) for the increase in embryo recovery with additional flushes are not known. It may be a result of the oxytocin administration or the additional uterine lavage procedure. Historical evidence has documented that approximately 10 to 30% of mares will become pregnant following an unsuccessful embryo collection attempt if no prostaglandins are administered. This suggests that some embryos remain within the reproductive tract (oviduct or uterus) after the flush procedure.

Alternatively, an additional flush procedure can be performed later the same day or the next day following a negative flush attempt. These delayed flushes are associated with an increased amount of cellular debris, but yield a viable embryo approximately 10% of the time.

Number of ET Cycles per Season

Donor mares are often bred and flushed during more than one estrous cycle per season in an attempt to obtain one or more pregnancies in recipient mares. Older subfertile mares may require more than one estrous cycle to recover an embryo and establish a single pregnancy in a recipient mare after transfer. In addition, a mare owner may want to obtain multiple pregnancies from a single donor mare in a single year.

The repetitive cycle of breeding and flushing may have deleterious effects on the uterine health of individual donor mares. Several studies have evaluated the effects of repeated embryo collection on either uterine health or embryo recovery rate. In general, repeated embryo collection seems to have little adverse effect on some individual donor mares, while evidence of increasing inflammation (i.e. fluid retained in the uterine lumen, increased white blood cells on uterine cytology, and increased numbers of lymphocytes present on endometrial biopsy) were present in other mares after 3 to 5 consecutive embryo transfer cycles.

It would be important to evaluate both the post-mating inflammatory response and the amount of debris in the fluid recovered during the embryo collection procedure to monitor the reproductive health of the mare. Individual mares that exhibit a progressive increase in either post-mating endometritis or debris in the uterine flush should be examined and may be candidates for time off from embryo transfer procedures.

It has been suggested that donor mares be limited to 5 cycles of breeding and flushing if signs of chronic PMIE are present and that the mare be allowed to carry her own foal to term every 3 to 4 years as a management procedure to optimize long-term uterine and cervical health.

Number of Ovulations

Ovulated oocytes may be fertilized in the oviduct and the developing embryo may eventually enter the uterus where it may be recovered. An increase in ovulation rate, either spontaneous or hormone induced, is generally associated with an increase in embryo collection rate per flush. In a recent study, an embryo was recovered on 46.8% of cycles (190 of 406) from client donor mares with a single ovulation and one or more embryos were recovered from 59.7% of cycles (43 of 72) from mares with two ovulations.

The sites of ovulation may influence embryo collection rate in mares that ovulate more than one follicle per cycle. Embryo recovery rate per ovulation in Argentinian polo horses that ovulated two or more follicles from the same ovary was less than the embryo recovery rate per ovulation in mares that ovulated follicles from opposite ovaries. It was hypothesized that ovum pickup by the oviduct may have been responsible for the decreased embryo recovery rate in mares with ipsilateral ovulations.

Clinical Expertise

Experience and development of sound technical skills are important in optimizing embryo recovery rates from mares. Problems encountered in embryo recovery are often associated with improper catheter placement, inadequate fluid recovery, poor flush technique, a fractious or anxious mare, and failure to identify an embryo in the search dish.

The embryo flush catheter should be passed through the cervix into the caudal uterine body before the cuff is inflated. The catheter should subsequently be gently retracted to 'lock' the cuff against the internal cervical os. Inflation of the cuff within the cervical canal may result in poor fluid recovery or failure of the catheter to remain in the reproductive tract of the mare. Insertion of the catheter too far up the uterus may result in inflation of the cuff within a uterine horn.

Ideally, all of the flush medium infused into the uterus should be recovered and passed through an embryo filter. Failure to recover fluid from the uterus may be associated with a decreased embryo recovery rate. Fluid recovery may be aided by massage of the uterus per rectum and administration of oxytocin (i.e. 10 to 20 units, intravenously). Monitoring fluid recovery into graduated cylinders can be of great importance. If fluid remains in the uterus, it is recommended that an ultrasound examination of the reproductive tract be performed to determine the location and volume of the residual fluid. The cuff can subsequently be deflated and the tip of the catheter advanced to a location within the fluid pocket. Additional flush media may have to be infused to restart the siphon effect and facilitate fluid recovery.

It is common practice to manipulate the catheter from outside the mare to aid in fluid recovery (i.e. to free the tip of the catheter if it was sucked up against the endometrium). However, if the catheter is aggressively manipulated, the endometrium may bleed from the irritation. Blood in the recovered fluid may interfere with the ability to identify an embryo. A gentle recovery technique should prevent the occurrence of bleeding associated with catheter manipulation. If blood is present in the fluid within the filter, it is recommended to rinse the filter with a large quantity of additional medium to dilute out the red blood cells by passing them through the filter.

Sedation of the mare during the flush procedure is at the option of the clinician. In our experience, sedation is not required for most mares. However, it may be beneficial to sedate young maiden mares, anxious mares and fractious mares to optimize the embryo recovery rate. Safety of the mare and personnel should be considered in addition to the efficiency and thoroughness of the flush procedure.

Recommended Reading

Allen WR, Wilsher S, Morris L, Crowhurst JS, Hillyer MH, Neal HN. Laparoscopic application of PGE2 to re-establish oviductal patency and fertility in infertile mares: a preliminary study. Equine Veterinary Journal 2006; 38: 454–459.

Ball BA, Little TV, Hillman RB, Woods GL. Pregnancy rates at Days 2 and 14 and estimated embryonic loss rates prior to day 14 in normal and subfertile mares. Theriogenology 1986; 26:611-619.

Bennett SD, Griffin RL, Rhoads WS. Surgical evaluation of oviduct disease and patency in the mare; Proceedings of the American Association of Equine Practitioners 2002; 48:347-349.

Carnevale EM, Coutinho da Silva MA, Panzani D, Stokes JE, Squires EL. Factors affecting the success of oocyte transfer in a clinical program for subfertile mares. Theriogenology; 2005; 64:519-527.

Hinrichs K. A simple technique that may improve the rate of embryo recovery on uterine flushing in mares. Theriogenology 1990; 33:937-942.

Ley WB, Bowen JM, Purswell BJ, Dascanio JJ, Parker NA, Bailey TL, DiGrassie WA. Modified technique to evaluate uterine tubal patency in the mare. Proceedings of the American Association of Equine Practitioners, AAEP 1998; 44:56-59.

Riera FL, Roldan JE, Hinrichs K. Patterns of embryo recovery in mares with unilateral and bilateral double ovulations. Anim Reprod Sci 2006; 94:398.

CHAPTER 8

EMBRYO HANDLING

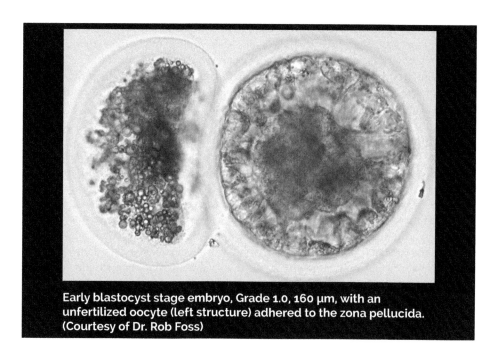

Early blastocyst stage embryo, Grade 1.0, 160 μm, with an
unfertilized oocyte (left structure) adhered to the zona pellucida.
(Courtesy of Dr. Rob Foss)

Technique

Once identified in the search dish, small to moderate sized embryos (i.e. 150 to 1,000 μm in diameter) are removed using a 0.25 ml semen straw attached to a 1.0 ml syringe via a syringe-straw connector (Figure 8-1). Larger embryos (i.e. > 1,000 μm in diameter) are removed using a 0.5 ml semen straw attached to a 1.0 ml syringe. Very large embryos are removed with a shortened artificial insemination pipette or other sterile device.

The embryo should be moved from the original search dish with as little fluid as possible and transferred through a series of wash steps to remove potential contaminants. Media used for washing can be embryo flush medium or commercial holding medium. It is recommended that the embryo be serially transferred through a minimum of 3 and up to 10 aliquots of wash medium. The wash medium can be a series of droplets within a small (60 mm) sterile petri dish (Figure 8-2) or can be medium placed into wells of a commercially available multi-well plate (Figure 8-3).

The goal of washing is to remove bacteria and cellular debris from the embryo, which otherwise may otherwise decrease pregnancy rate after transfer. Occasionally an embryo is recovered with debris adherent to the zona pellucida (Figure 8-4). In most instances, a majority of the debris can be removed by sequential washing steps. However, in some cases the debris cannot be removed completely and the embryo will need to be transferred into the recipient mare. In this situation, it may be prudent to administer antimicrobial agents to the recipient mare systemically to help decrease the possibility that the recipient mare will develop bacterial endometritis and subsequently not remain pregnant. The donor mare in that instance should be examined by culture and cytology to determine if she has a uterine infection.

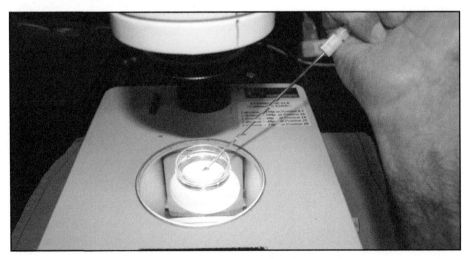

Figure 8-1. Transferring an embryo from one petri dish to another using a 0.25 ml semen straw attached to a 1.0 ml syringe.

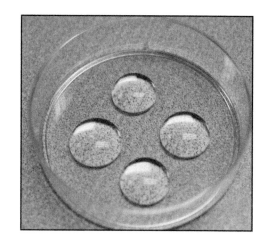

Figure 8-2. Droplets of holding medium within a 60 mm petri dish used to wash embryos.

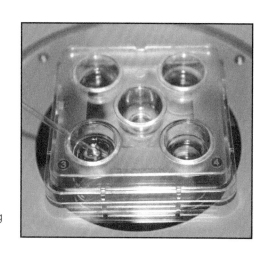

Figure 8-3. Multi-well plate containing holding medium to wash embryos.

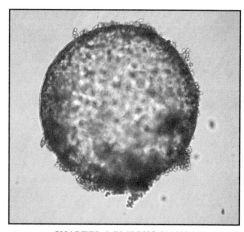

Figure 8-4. Blastocyst stage embryo with debris adherent to the zona pellucida.

The embryo can be transferred immediately or maintained in holding medium at room temperature (20° to 22° C) for 2 to 4 hours prior to transfer. If the interval from collection to transfer is of a longer duration it may be beneficial to cool the embryo to approximately 5 to 8° C in a passive cooling system (i.e. Equitainer®, Hamilton Research, Inc., South Hamilton, MA). Controlled clinical trials to critically evaluate the duration of storage at room temperature in commercial holding media and associated pregnancy rates have not been reported.

Recommended Reading

Squires EL, GE Seidel Jr. Collection and transfer of equine embryos. Colorado State University Animal Reproduction and Biotechnology Laboratory Bulletin No. 8, 1995; 64 pp.

Stringfellow DA. Recommendations for the sanitary handling of in-vivo-derived embryos. In: Stringfellow DA and Seidel SM (eds), Manual of the International Embryo Transfer Society. Third edition. IETS, Savoy, Illinois; 1998, pp. 79-84.

CHAPTER 9

EVALUATION OF EQUINE EMBRYOS

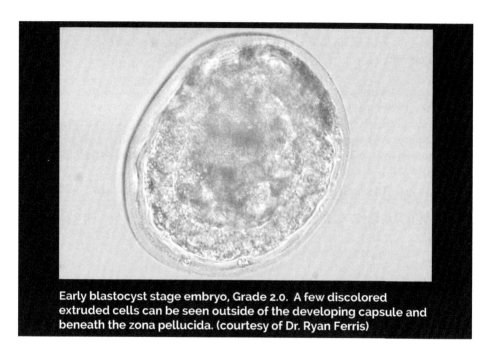

Early blastocyst stage embryo, Grade 2.0. A few discolored extruded cells can be seen outside of the developing capsule and beneath the zona pellucida. (courtesy of Dr. Ryan Ferris)

Introduction

The ability to accurately evaluate developmental stage, assess quality, and determine size of an equine embryo is critical to the success of an embryo transfer program. It is also important to be able to differentiate between an embryo, an unfertilized oocyte (UFO), and non-embryonic structures that may be recovered during an embryo flush procedure.

It is recommended that a consistent method be used for embryo evaluation and that an accurate log be maintained of all embryos and subsequent transfer success. It is also recommended that photographs be captured of all embryos, if possible. Decisions on selection of an appropriate recipient mare, prognosis for transfer success, and ability to determine if an embryo can be successfully cryopreserved are dependent on an accurate embryo evaluation.

Embryo evaluation usually takes only a few moments to perform and can provide valuable information as to the probability that a given embryo may survive after transfer. The primary goal is to determine embryo quality, but the evaluation may also identify embryos with significant abnormalities, differentiate unfertilized oocytes from small embryos, and determine if the developmental stage is consistent with embryo age.

Embryo Development and Morphologic Characteristics

Morphologic features of equine embryos must be understood in order to evaluate developmental stages and assess embryo quality (Table 9-1).

After fertilization, a series of cleavage divisions transforms the one-cell zygote into 2-cell, 4-cell and 8-cell stage embryos. Each individual cell of the embryo, called blastomeres, is maintained within the outer acellular zona pellucida. The developing embryo is at the morula stage when 16 or more blastomeres are present. A gap, termed the perivitelline space, may be present between the blastomeres and the zona pellucida of a compact morula. As embryonic development continues, the morula transitions into a blastocyst as cell divisions proceed and a small fluid filled cavity or blastocoele begins to form within the center of the embryo. The blastocyst consists of an outer rim of trophoblast cells and a distinct inner cell mass embedded within the wall of trophoblast cells. The trophoblast layer will eventually form the placenta and the inner cell mass will form the embryo proper. An equine embryo is usually at the morula or early blastocyst stage of development when it first enters the uterus. Trophoblast cells of in vivo maturing embryos produce an acellular glycoprotein coat called the capsule in between the trophoblast layer and the outer zona pellucida. The capsule is unique to equine embryos and can be observed microscopically as a pale-yellow refractile layer underneath the zona pellucida. As the blastocyst expands, the zona pellucida becomes thinner and eventually is shed. The equine embryo does not "hatch" from its zona pellucida like ruminant embryos. After the zona pellucida has been lost, the capsule is the only membrane surrounding the embryo.

Table 9-1.
Normal structures associated with the equine embryo.

Embryonic Structure	Description
Blastocoele	Fluid-filled cavity surrounded by a single layer of trophoblast cells of the blastocyst stage embryo
Blastomere	One of the cells comprising the early embryo
Capsule	Acellular glycoprotein envelope produced by trophoblast cells; initially located between the trophectoderm and zona pellucida; becomes the outer protective layer after the zona is shed; unique to the horse
Inner cell mass	Cluster of blastomeres that will differentiate to form the embryo proper and eventually the fetus
Perivitelline space	Potential space between the blastomeres of a morula-stage embryo or the trophoblast cells of a blastocyst stage embryo and the zona pellucida
Trophoblast	Layer of extraembryonic ectodermal tissue that differentiates during formation of the blastocyst stage embryo and surrounds the blastocoele cavity; eventually forms the chorion and amnion
Zona pellucida	Noncellular glycoprotein coat surrounding the oocyte and early embryo; eventually thins and is shed as the equine embryo expands

Embryo Assessment

A good quality microscope, with an eyepiece micrometer for measurement of embryo diameter, is essential for a proper embryo evaluation (see Chapter 6). It is recommended that the evaluation determine developmental stage, quality score or grade, and size (μm). Additional comments should be recorded for quantity and character of debris in the flush, presence of debris or cells attached to the embryo and morphological abnormalities of the embryo.

Developmental Stages

The developmental stage of an embryo is normally directly related to age or the number of days after ovulation. Morula or early blastocyst stage equine embryos enter the uterus between 130 to 142 hours after ovulation. Oviductal transport through the isthmus and the uterotubular junction is dependent on production of prostaglandin E_2 (PGE_2) from a viable embryo.

Morula stage embryos are 150 to 200 μm in diameter, have a thick zona pellucida and large distinct blastomeres that provide a "scalloped" or "serrated" appearance to the outer edge of the mass of cells (Figure 9-1). Further cleavage divisions and tight junctional complexes between blastomeres leads to formation of a compact morula, with a perivitelline space visible between the embryo and zona pellucida (Figure 9-2). The morula may be spherical or slightly oval in shape and will roll on manipulation.

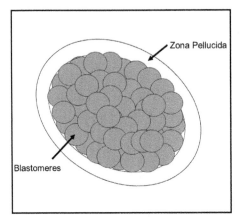
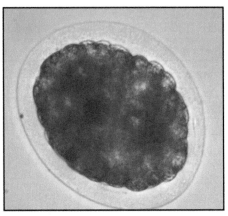

Figure 9-1. Morula stage equine embryo (Grade 1). Note the thick zona pellucida and large blastomeres.

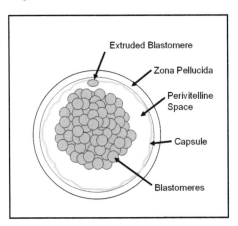
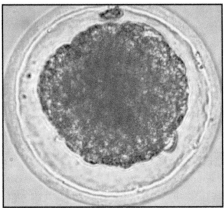

Figure 9-2. Compact morula stage embryo (Grade 1). Note the refractile capsule beneath the zona pellucida, large perivitelline space, and a single extruded blastomere.

Early blastocyst stage embryos are 150 to 250 μm in diameter or approximately the same overall size as a morula, have a thick zona pellucida, but are comprised of a larger number of smaller cells (Figure 9-3). Secretion of fluid produced by the blastomeres leads to formation of the blastocoele cavity, a small fluid-filled pocket or space within the embryo, which is the hallmark of the blastocyst stage embryo. As viewed through the microscope, this space often appears slightly darker than the surrounding cells and the edges are difficult to distinguish. The perivitelline space is usually minimal or absent.

Blastocyst stage embryos are 150 to 300 μm in diameter and develop following continued cellular division and fluid secretion, yielding a distinct trophoblast layer surrounding a blastocoele cavity (Figure 9-4). A cluster of cells that protrudes slightly into the blastocoele is the developing inner cell mass. The trophoblast layer will form the placenta and the inner cell mass will form the embryo proper and eventually the fetus. An acellular capsule, unique to the horse, begins to form

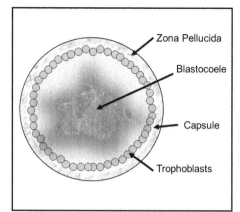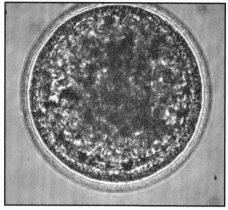

Figure 9-3. Early blastocyst stage equine embryo (Grade 1). Note the thinner zona pellucida, capsule and small blastocoele cavity.

between the trophoblast layer and the thin zona pellucida 6 to 7 days after ovulation and disappears by day 23. The capsule is formed from glycoproteins produced by trophoblast cells, with possible contributions from maternal tissue. As viewed through the microscope, the capsule appears irregular, refractile, and slightly yellowish in color. The precise functions of the capsule are not well established. It may be important in facilitation of embryo migration, physical protection of the embryo, and prevention of immunological recognition during early embryonic development.

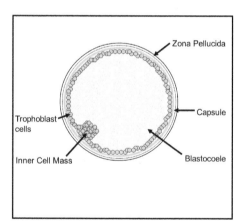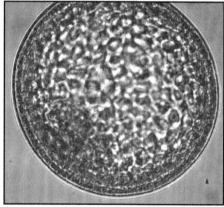

Figure 9-4. Blastocyst stage equine embryo (Grade 1). Note the thin zona pellucida, blastocoele cavity and distinct inner cell mass.

Expanded blastocyst stage embryos are 300 to > 1,000 μm in diameter and result from rapid expansion of the embryo on day 7 post-ovulation (Figure 9-5). A large blastocoele cavity is surrounded by a thin layer of trophoblast cells which are small and uniform in appearance. The zona pellucida becomes progressively thinner as the embryo increases in diameter and is eventually shed. Subsequently, the outer surface of the embryo is covered only by the capsule. The capsule may be tightly adherent to the embryo or slightly detached (Figure 9-6). Embryos recovered on day 8 may be more than double in size as compared to embryos recovered on day 7.

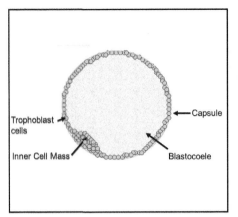 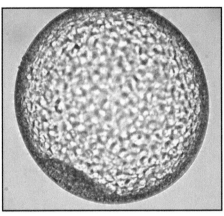

Figure 9-5. Expanded blastocyst stage embryo (Grade 1). The zona pellucida has been shed and the capsule is tightly surrounding the embryo.

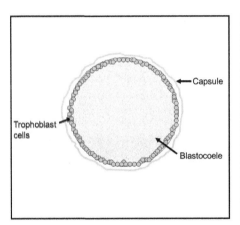 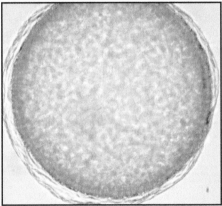

Figure 9-6. Large expanded blastocyst stage embryo (Grade 1). Note the capsule outside of the trophoblast layer. No inner cell mass is visible on this view.

Unfertilized Oocytes

Unfertilized oocytes (UFOs) are typically 125 to 150 μm in diameter, round or oval in shape, but are flat and do not roll when manipulated (Figure 9-7). The zona pellucida is thick and the cytoplasm of this single-cell may degenerate and fragment and lead to a somewhat similar appearance as a morula stage embryo (Figure 9-8).

In contrast to an embryo, an unfertilized oocyte is generally retained within the oviduct near the ampulla-isthmus junction. However, unfertilized oocytes are recovered during 3.6% to 12.9% of embryo collection attempts. In most such instances, the UFO is transported down the isthmus and through the utero-tubular junction along with a viable embryo. Consequently, detection of a UFO in a uterine flush is usually indicative of the presence of an embryo. If an embryo is not located in the search dish, it may be beneficial to re-flush the mare immediately or the following morning.

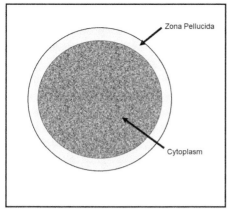
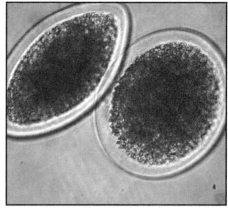

Figure 9-7. A pair of unfertilized oocytes. Note the thick zona pellucida and lack of individual blastomeres in these single-cell oocytes.

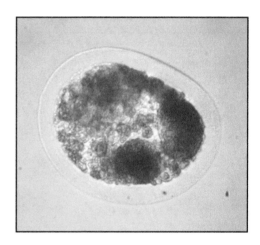

Figure 9-8. Degenerated unfertilized oocyte. Note that the fragmented cytoplasm of this single-cell structure may look like blastomeres of a morula stage embryo.

Non-Embryonic Structures

Cellular debris, urine crystals, organic material, and other debris are sometimes recovered during embryo collection attempts and may cause confusion on the part of the clinician (Figures 9-9 through 9-11). Differentiation of non-embryos from a morula or early blastocyst stage embryo is critically important and adherence to the principles of embryo evaluation will usually lead to a correct identification. First, early embryos are surrounded by a distinct thick zona pellucida. Non-embryonic structures recovered from uterine washings do not have an investment or outer coating similar to a zona pellucida. Second, early embryos are spherical in shape which allows an embryo to be "rolled" easily along the floor of a Petri dish when the dish is swirled or in response to pressure from a briefly applied bolus of medium. In contrast, most non-embryonic structures are not spherical and do not "roll". Determination of the size of the structure will also help with differentiation. Early uterine stage embryos will typically be 180 to 250 µm in diameter. A majority of confusing, slightly spherical non-embryonic structures are only 50 to 100 µm in diameter.

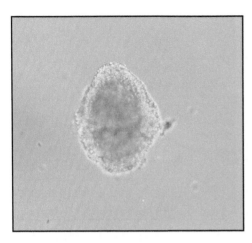

Figure 9-9. Mass of non-embryonic cells 180 µm in diameter recovered during an embryo collection attempt. Note lack of zona pellucida. The structure was flat and did not roll on manipulation.

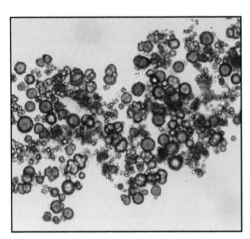

Figure 9-10. Mass of non-embryonic structures <150 µm in diameter recovered during an embryo collection attempt. Note lack of zona pellucida.

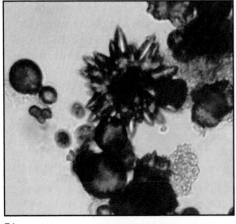

Figure 9-11. Urine crystals and small (50 µm) spherical structures recovered during an embryo collection attempt.

If one is still unsure about the status of a possible embryo that is intended for shipment to an embryo transfer referral center, it may be prudent to contact the center for a consultation. If your microscope is equipped with a digital camera, a photograph can be emailed to the referral center for evaluation and a second opinion. If that is not possible, or the diagnosis is still in doubt, it may be best to package the unknown structure and ship it to the transfer center for a final diagnosis. It is recommended that a note indicating the size, shape and other features of the unknown structure be included within the shipment container.

Embryo Grading

Evaluation of embryo morphology is used to assign a quality score or grade to an embryo. Embryo grade is positively correlated to pregnancy rate after transfer and inversely correlated to pregnancy loss rate between days 16 and 50. An accurate assessment of embryo morphology may be performed rapidly, but requires training and a stereomicroscope with good optics at 10x to 50x. Morphologic characteristics considered when assigning a grade are presented in Table 9-2; embryos of various grades are presented in Figures 9-12 through 9-17.

A 4-point grading system may be used to evaluate equine embryos (Table 9-3). In this system, unfertilized oocytes are not part of the scoring system since they are not embryos, and both degenerated and dead embryos are included in Grade 4. Similar grading systems have been used to evaluate *in vitro* produced equine embryos. Subclassifications of Grades are often used in practice to describe embryos with a morphologic grade midway between two defined scores (i.e. Grade 1.5, 2.5, or 3.5).

Table 9-2.
Morphologic characteristics used to evaluate quality of equine embryos.

Characteristic
Developmental stage relative to embryo age
Size of embryo relative to embryo age
Shape of embryo (spherical, oval, collapsed, etc.)
Thickness of zona pellucida
Uniformity of blastomeres (size, color, structure)
Presence/absence of extruded or degenerated blastomeres
Compactness of blastomeres
Degree of cytoplasmic granulation or fragmentation
Presence/absence and size of perivitelline space
Evidence of dehydration or shrinkage of embryo
Presence/absence of abnormalities of the blastocoele
Presence/absence of damage to the zona pellucida or capsule

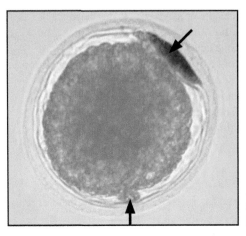

Figure 9-12. Grade 2 early blastocyst stage embryo; note extruded blastomeres (arrows).

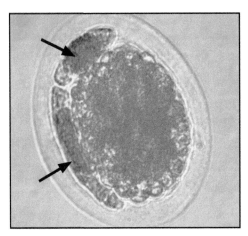

Figure 9-13. Grade 3 morula stage embryo; note large percentage of extruded blastomeres (arrows).

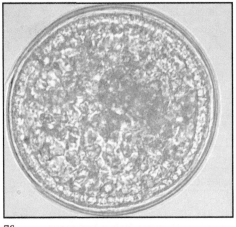

Figure 9-14. Grade 1 blastocyst stage embryo 300 µm in diameter. No morphologic abnormalities are present in this embryo.

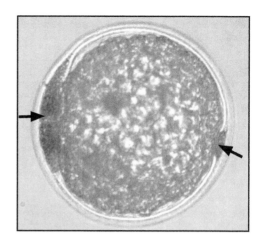

Figure 9-15. Grade 2 blastocyst 220 µm in diameter. Note the extruded blastomeres (arrows), occasional discolored cell and slight shrinkage from zona pellucida.

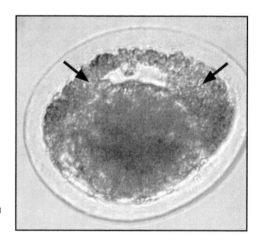

Figure 9-16. Grade 3 morula stage embryo 200 µm in diameter. Note the high proportion of extruded blastomeres (arrows) and discoloration of remaining cell mass.

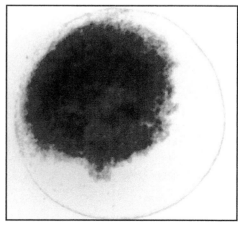

Figure 9-17. Grade 4 embryo. Note the complete degeneration of the embryo within the capsule.

Table 9-3.
Embryo grade assignment based on a 4-point system. Modified from the Manual of the International Embryo Transfer Society (IETS).

Grade	Comment	Description
1	Excellent	No significant abnormalities observed; symmetrical and spherical in shape; cells of uniform size, color and texture; size and developmental stage appropriate for age post-ovulation
2	Good	Minor imperfections, such as a few extruded blastomeres; slight irregularities in shape, size, color, or texture; limited separation between trophoblast layer and zona pellucida or capsule
3	Poor	Moderate level of imperfections, such as a larger percentage of extruded or degenerated blastomeres; partial collapse of blastocoele; or moderate shrinkage of trophoblast from zona pellucida or capsule
4	Degenerate or Dead	Severe problems easily identified, such as a high percentage of extruded blastomeres, complete collapse of blastocoele, rupture of zona pellucida, or complete degeneration and embryonic death

Occasionally a normal equine embryo recovered at day 7 postovulation is observed to have a few cells or even a spermatozoon attached to the zona pellucida (Figures 9-18 through 9-21). These cells may be cumulus cells still attached to the zona pellucida and are of little to no clinical consequence.

Adherence of multiple clumps of cells or other material to the zona pellucida may be a sign of endometritis in the donor mare or contamination of the flush procedure. Affected embryos should be washed as thoroughly as possible and consideration should be given to treatment of the recipient mare with broad spectrum antibiotics beginning at the time of transfer and continuing for the subsequent 5 to 7 days. The presence of debris attached to the outside of the embryo does not influence the assignment of grade. Grade is assigned based solely on morphologic characteristics of the embryo. The presence of external debris is clinically important and is recorded as additional comments.

The vast majority of embryos collected from donor mares are good to excellent in quality (Table 9-4). This is likely due to the selective transport of viable embryos through the oviduct. Poor quality embryos, dead embryos, and unfertilized oocytes are likely retained in the oviduct. Practitioners are faced with a decision when an embryo of poor quality is recovered, as transfer success of Grade 3 and 4 embryos is significantly lower than that of Grade 1 or 2 embryos and embryonic loss rate is higher. However, one certainty is that an embryo has no chance of survival if it is not transferred. It is recommended that all embryos be transferred, regardless of grade, if a recipient mare is available.

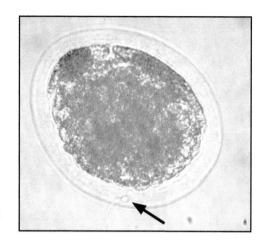

Figure 9-18. Grade 2 morula stage embryo with a sperm in zona pellucida (arrow).

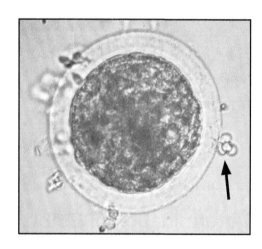

Figure 9-19. Grade 1 early blastocyst stage embryo. Note cumulus cells adhering to zona pellucida (arrow).

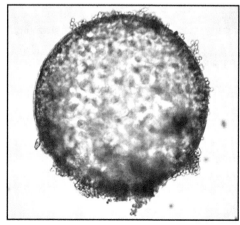

Figure 9-20. Blastocyst stage embryo with debris adherent to outside of zona pellucida.

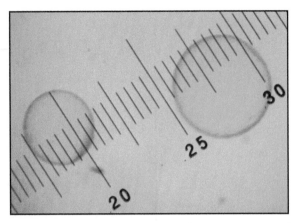

Figure 9-21. Measurement of embryo diameter using an eyepiece micrometer. Two expanded blastocyst stage embryos are visible.

Table 9-4.
Quality score (grade) of 623 embryos collected in a clinical embryo transfer program.

Embryo Grade	Embryos	
	Number	(%)
1.0 to 1.5	470	(75.4%)
2.0 to 2.5	125	(20.1%)
3.0 to 3.5	26	(4.2%)
4.0	2	(0.3%)
Total	623	(100%)

Determination of Embryo Size

An important, but sometimes overlooked, component of the embryo examination is determination of embryo size. Measurement of embryo size is used in conjunction with embryonic stage in evaluating development relative to age. An accurate measurement is also critical when deciding whether or not to cryopreserve an embryo. To date, cryopreservation of equine embryos is most successful on good quality, morula to early blastocyst stage embryos less than 300 μm in diameter.

In practice, a calibrated eyepiece micrometer is the easiest way to obtain an accurate measurement of embryo size (See Figure 9-21). The final size determination is based on a calibration scale taking into account the overall magnification used to obtain the measurement. It is generally sufficient to record in microns (μm) a single value for embryo diameter, measured from the outside of the zona pellucida at the widest part of the embryo. Diameter and embryonic stage are used to evaluate developmental competence relative to embryo age. Alternatively, an electronic caliper can be used if a camera and computer is attached to the microscope (Figure 9-22).

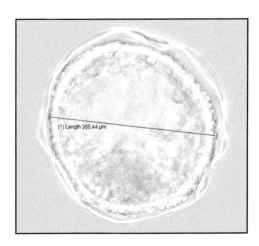

Figure 9-22. Measurement of embryo diameter using electronic calipers.

Small for Gestational Age (SFGA) Embryos

Recovery of an embryo that is smaller than expected and/or of an earlier developmental stage than expected is not unusual when performing an embryo collection attempt on an older mare or a mare that has been bred with frozen semen. Recovery of a SFGA embryo may reflect delayed embryonic development, inadequate oviductal or uterine environment, or other factors. Recognition that an embryo is delayed in development is important, as pregnancy rates may be optimized if the embryo is transferred into a mare that is synchronized relative to embryonic development, rather than ovulation day of the donor mare. In addition, embryonic loss rate may be higher for a SFGA embryo if a pregnancy is established in a recipient mare after transfer.

Photographs of Embryos

Practitioners are encouraged to photograph all embryos prior to transfer. Photographs provide a permanent record of embryo stage, grade, and size. Embryo photographs also provide an excellent mechanism by which to train new staff so that embryo evaluation procedures are standardized throughout the practice.

Recommended Reading

McCue PM, DeLuca CA, Ferris RA, Wall JJ. How to evaluate equine embryos. Proceedings, American Association of Equine Practitioners 2009; 55: 252-256.

McKinnon AO, Squires EL. Morphologic assessment of the equine embryo. J Am Vet Med Assoc 1988; 192:401-406.

Robertson I, Nelson RE. Certification and identification of the embryo. In: Stringfellow DA and Seidel SM (eds), Manual of the International Embryo Transfer Society. Third edition. IETS, Savoy, Illinois; 1998, pp. 103-116.

Vanderwall DK. Early embryonic development and evaluation of equine embryo viability. Vet Clin North Am Equine Pract 1996; 12:61-83.

Squires EL, Seidel Jr., GE. Collection and transfer of equine embryos. Colorado State University Bulletin No. 08. 1995. pp. 18-23.

CHAPTER 10

COOLED-TRANSPORTED EMBRYOS

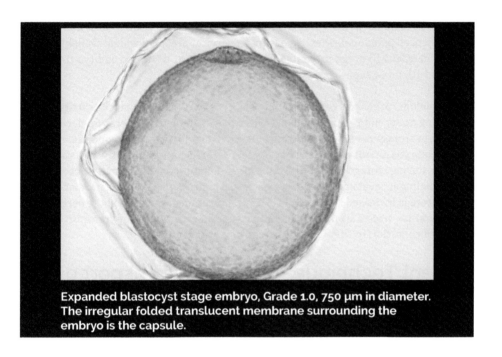

Expanded blastocyst stage embryo, Grade 1.0, 750 μm in diameter. The irregular folded translucent membrane surrounding the embryo is the capsule.

Introduction

Cooled-transport of equine embryos is now a routine procedure in the equine industry. Progress in development of commercial complete holding media and passive cooling systems have simplified the process.

The major advantages of transporting embryos are that 1) donor mares can be maintained and managed at home; transport is only necessary if an embryo is recovered, 2) cost of transport of an embryo is significantly less than transport of a mare, 3) housing recipient mares at specialized centers eliminates the need to maintain a recipient herd at every breeding farm; recipients are often best managed by experienced personnel, 4) embryo transfer services are more widely available to mare owners, and 5) pregnancy rates are usually better at dedicated embryo transfer facilities with more experienced personnel.

The physiologic principles behind cooling embryos for short term storage are based on slowing down embryo metabolism. A decrease in ambient temperature during short-term storage results in a slowing of embryo metabolism. Consequently, equine embryos do not advance in developmental stage or significantly increase in diameter during storage at 5° C. The inhibition of embryo metabolism that occurs during cooling is reversible, as embryos increase in diameter when the incubation temperature is increased back to 37° C. Clinically, cooling provides a short period (i.e. < 24 hours) for *in vitro* storage during which time an embryo may be transported from the site of collection to the site of transfer into a recipient.

Current Technique for Cooled-Transport of Equine Embryos

Materials required

1. Commercial Embryo Holding Medium
2. 5-ml sterile plastic tube with screw or snap cap (Figure 10-1)
3. 50-ml sterile centrifuge tube with screw cap
4. Parafilm® sealing film

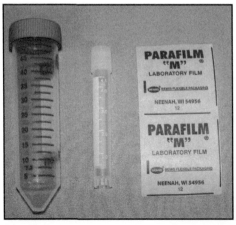

Figure 10-1. 50-ml conical tube, 5-ml vial and Parafilm® for cooled-storage of equine embryos.

5. Passive cooling device (i.e. Equitainer®)

6. Embryo flush media (50 mls) – saved prior to embryo flush

Directions for packaging an embryo for shipment

1. Allow the embryo holding medium to warm to 37° C.

2. Fill the 5-ml plastic tube with approximately 4.5 mls of warmed holding medium.

3. Carefully transfer the embryo (after washing through a minimum of 3 to 4 drops of holding medium) into the plastic tube. Rinse out the transfer straw and observe rinse medium under microscope to ensure that the embryo was properly transferred.

4. Slowly add more medium until the 5-ml tube is full. Fix the cap securely in place. Seal the tube with Parafilm® sealing film.

5. Fill the 50-ml centrifuge tube with the saved flush medium.

6. Place the 5-ml tube containing the embryo into the 50-ml centrifuge tube. Attach the cap of the centrifuge tube securely in place and seal with Parafilm® (Figure 10-2).

7. Load the 50-ml tube containing the embryo into the passive cooling device (Figure 10-3)

8. Insert appropriate documentation, including a description of the embryo (i.e. developmental stage, grade and size).

9. Ship the container to the embryo transfer referral center by counter-to-counter airline delivery (preferred) or overnight courier service.

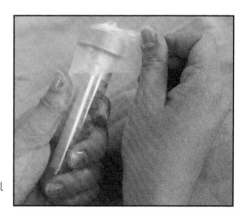

Figure 10-2. Application of Parafilm® to seal the 50-ml conical tube.

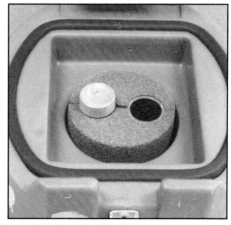

Figure 10-3. 50-ml conical tube containing an embryo within a commercial passive cooling container.

Directions for receiving and handling a shipped embryo

1. Open the container in a clean laboratory space and review documentation.
2. Have embryo holding medium available to wash embryo or rinse plastic tube.
3. Open centrifuge tube and remove 5-ml tube containing embryo.
4. Gently invert the 5-ml tube several times.
5. Remove cap from 5-ml tube, place cap with open end up on counter top and add several drops of holding medium into cap.
6. Pour contents of 5-ml tube into a sterile 60 mm Petri dish.
7. Add several drops of holding medium into empty 5-ml tube and set aside.
8. Search Petri dish for embryo.
9. If the embryo is not immediately visible, rinse the cap and the 5-ml tube several times with holding medium. Embryos occasionally will stick to the plastic tube or cap.
10. Wash the embryo through a minimum of 3 to 4 drops of holding medium prior to transfer. Ideally, the medium used to wash the embryo should be the same as the medium used for cooled storage. Occasionally some shrinkage of a cooled-transported embryo may be observed (Figure 10-4 and 10-5).

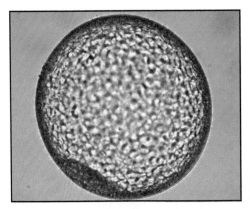

Figure 10-4. Fresh day 7.5 expanded blastocyst prior to transfer.

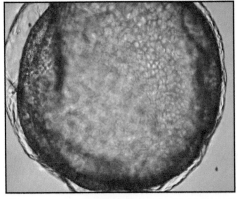

Figure 10-5. Cooled day 8 expanded blastocyst exhibiting mild shrinkage or dehydration. The capsule is visible surrounding the embryo.

Pregnancy Rates in a Commercial Embryo Transfer Program

Quality scores or grade for 622 fresh and cooled equine embryos evaluated immediately prior to transfer at Colorado State University are presented in Table 10-1. The highest percentage of Grade 1 embryos (81.2%) occurred with fresh embryos. Cooled storage for approximately 12 to 24 hours, for counter-to-counter or overnight courier service, respectively, was associated with lower quality scores.

Table 10-1.
Quality score for equine embryos immediately prior to transfer (number of embryos and percentage for each grade). Embryos were either transferred immediately after collection (fresh) or after having been cooled for approximately 12 hours (counter-to-counter transport) or 24 hours (overnight courier transport).

Embryo Storage	Grade 1	Grade 2	Grades 3 + 4
Fresh	303 (81.2%)	61 (16.4%)	9 (2.4%)
Counter-to-Counter	159 (68.8%)	57 (24.7%)	15 (6.5%)
Overnight Courier	8 (44.4%)	7 (38.9%)	3 (16.7%)

Pregnancy Rate – Fresh vs. Cooled Embryos

Pregnancy rates are not different following transfer of fresh Grade 1 embryos than following transfer of Grade 1 embryos that had been cooled and transported for 12 to 24 hours in a passive cooling system (Table 10-2). A decrease in pregnancy rate was noted following transfer of lesser quality embryos that had been cooled and transported.

There was no significant difference in pregnancy loss rate between days 16 and 50 for embryos transferred immediately after collection and cooled embryos transferred after same day or overnight delivery.

The incidence of "empty trophoblastic vesicle" (ETV) formation may be slightly higher after cooled storage of an equine embryo as compared to an embryo that was transferred immediately after collection.

Table 10-2.
Day 16 pregnancy rates for equine embryos by Grade and status (fresh vs. cooled).

Embryo Grade	Fresh Embryos		Cooled Embryos	
	(n)	Pregnancy Rate	(n)	Pregnancy Rate
1	639	76.3%	232	76.2%
2	53	79.2%	48	60.4%
3 & 4	80	56.2%	30	53.3%

References

Carnevale EM, Squires EL, McKinnon AO. Comparison of Ham's F-10 with CO_2 or Hepes buffer for storage of equine embryos at 5° C for 24 h. J Anim Sci 1987;65:1775-1781.

McCue PM, DeLuca CA, Wall JJ. Cooled transported embryo technology. In: Equine Reproduction. Second Edition. McKinnon AO, EL Squires, WE Vaala, DD Varner (Eds). Wiley-Blackwell, Ames, Iowa. 2011, pp 2880-2886.

Moussa M, Tremoleda JL, Duchamp G, Bruyas J-F, Colenbrander B, Bevers MM, Daels PF. Evaluation of viability and apoptosis in horse embryos stored under different conditions at 5° C. Theriogenology 2004;61:921-932.

CHAPTER 11

CRYOPRESERVATION OF EQUINE EMBRYOS

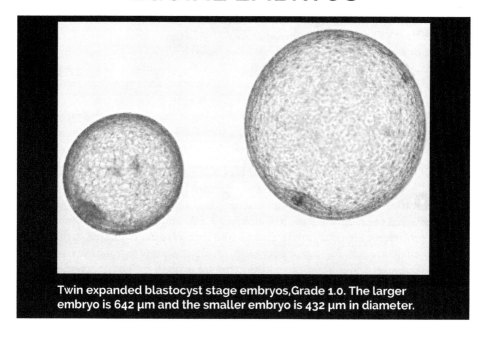

Twin expanded blastocyst stage embryos,Grade 1.0. The larger embryo is 642 µm and the smaller embryo is 432 µm in diameter.

Introduction

The birth of the first calf from a frozen-thawed embryo was in 1973, but it was not until 1982 that scientists in Japan reported the birth of the first foal from a frozen-thawed equine embryo. The following year Colorado State University produced 2 foals from 4 frozen-thawed embryos transferred to recipient mares. Since that time there have been numerous studies evaluating various methods for long-term storage of equine embryos. However, only recently cryopreservation of equine embryos has gained popularity and become a viable clinical procedure.

Reasons for cryopreserving equine embryos include:
1. Preservation of genetics of a valuable mare.
2. Import or export of embryos.
3. Minimization of the number of recipients needed for an embryo transfer program.
4. Multiple embryos may be collected after superovulation and stored for later transfer.
5. Allows for collection of embryos later in a breeding season and transfer early the following breeding season for early foal production.

Effect of Embryo Diameter on Cryopreservation

Historically, acceptable pregnancy rates after transfer have been achieved following cryopreservation of embryos < 300 µm in diameter, whereas poor pregnancy rates have resulted from cryopreservation of embryos > 300 µm. Consequently, embryo recovery procedures are usually performed 6.5 to 7.0 days after ovulation in order to collect small embryos for cryopreservation. An alternative is to flush the donor mare 8.0 days after administration of hCG to induce ovulation. The latter technique is dependent on ovulation occurring approximately 36 hours after hCG administration which is not always consistent. There is considerable variation between individual mares in the response to hCG. It is advisable to monitor individual mares once or twice daily to narrow the time of ovulation to optimize the odds of harvesting a small morula or early blastocyst stage embryo for cryopreservation. In addition, embryonic development may be different in older mares, mares inseminated postovulation or mares inseminated with frozen semen.

A recent study reported success with cryopreservation of large embryos (> 400 µm) after removal of blastocoele fluid, being vitrified in ethylene glycol and warmed/thawed in a sucrose solution.

Methods of Embryo Cryopreservation
Slow Cool Method

The first foals produced from frozen-thawed embryos were by a method similar to that used in the cattle industry termed "slow cooling", which required a programmable controlled rate freezer. Small embryos (< 220 µm in diameter) were washed by transfer through five successive drops of modified Dulbecco's phosphate buffered saline with 5% heat-treated fetal calf serum. Glycerol was added as the cryoprotectant in two steps: 5% v\v in PBS for 10 minutes followed by 10% glycerol for 20 to 30 minutes.

Embryos were loaded into 0.25 ml straws and placed in a programmable freezer for cooling. Embryos were cooled from room temperature to -6° C at 4° per minute and then seeded by contacting the straw with stainless steel forceps that had been previously cooled in liquid nitrogen. Samples were held at -6° C for 15 minutes and then cooled at 0.3° C per minute to -34 to -35° C before being plunged into liquid nitrogen.

Frozen embryos were thawed by immersing the straw in a water bath at 37° C and gently agitated until all the ice within the straw had melted (30 to 60 seconds). The embryos were recovered from the straws and placed in fresh 10% glycerol in PBS with 5% fetal calf serum. The cryoprotectant was diluted by transferring the embryo through six successively drops of less concentrated glycerol solutions. An equilibration time of 10 minutes was allowed for each dilution step.

Cryopreservation of equine embryos using the slow cool method has resulted in acceptable pregnancy rates with small embryos. However, the technique requires expensive equipment and takes approximately an hour and a half to freeze an embryo.

Vitrification Method

Vitrification is an ultrarapid freezing process for cryopreservation that does not require specialized equipment. Embryos are exposed to high concentrations of permeating cryoprotectants that prevents ice crystal formation upon exposure to liquid nitrogen resulting in a "glass- like formation" within the embryo. Another advantage of vitrification is that the embryo can be rapidly warmed (thawed) within the straw and the straw loaded into a Cassou gun for direct transfer into the recipient mare.

Vitrification kits are available from several companies. The kits contain a series of three vials of vitrification solutions, a vial of diluent (i.e. galactose) and instructions. Vitrification solutions contain different concentrations of glycerol and ethylene glycol (Table 11-1).

Table 11-1.
An example of cryoprotectants in one vitrification protocol.

Solution	Glycerol	Ethylene Glycol	Galactose
1	1.4 M	--	--
2	1.4 M	3.6 M	--
3	3.4 M	4.6 M	--
Diluent	--	--	0.5 M

A practical technique for vitrification of small (< 300 μm) equine embryos is as follows:
Initial Preparation Steps:
1. Identify and wash embryo through multiple drops of commercial holding medium.
2. Place embryo in a small (35 mm diameter) petri dish containing commercial holding medium. The embryo should be vitrified as soon as possible after collection.

Vitrification Procedure:

1. Prepare a petri dish (100 mm diameter) with 5 labeled areas for the vitrification solutions (Figure 11-1). One area for solution-1, one area for solution-2, one area for solution-3 and two areas for diluent.

2. Set a timer to 5 minutes.

3. Move 200 µl of solution-1 to the designated spot on the petri dish.

4. Transfer embryo from holding medium using a 10 or 20 µl pipetter with the smallest volume of holding medium possible (i.e. set the pipetter to 1 µl).

5. Start timer immediately (5 minute countdown).

6. With about 1 minute remaining on the timer, transfer 200 µl of VS-2 into the appropriately labeled area of the petri dish.

7. After 5 minutes, move the embryo from solution 1 to solution 2 with minimum volume (1 µl) using the pipetter.

8. Start timer immediately (5 minute countdown).

9. With about 1 minute left.

    i. Transfer 90 µl of diluent solution containing galactose into each of the 2 designated spots on the petri dish

    ii. Transfer 30 µl of solution 3 into the designated spot

    iii. Set timer for 1 minute.

10. After 5 minutes in solution 2, move the embryo to solution 3. The exposure time to solution 3 is extremely important. Too long of an exposure in solution 3 can be toxic to the embryo.

11. Start timer (1 minute countdown).

12. Immediately:

    i. Draw up first diluent solution drop (90 µl) into a non-irradiated polyvinyl chloride 0.25 ml straw.

    ii. Add an air gap (5-10 µl).

    iii. Draw up solution 3 drop (30 µl) containing the embryo.

    iv. Add an air gap (5 to10 µl).

    v. Draw up the remaining (2nd) diluent solution drop (90 µl) until the initial fluid contacts the straw plug.

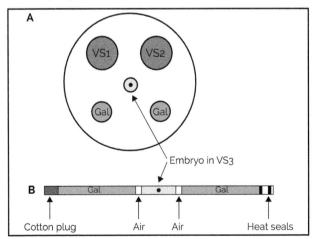

Figure 11-1. Petri dish prepared for vitrification of an embryo (From Carnevale, 2004). VS1, VS2 and VS3 refer to solutions 1, 2 and 3 respectively.

13. Plug the open end of the 0.25 ml straw with a Straw Adaptor and attach the other end of the adaptor to an appropriately labeled 0.5 ml straw. The 0.5 ml straw should contain information such as donor mare name, embryo collection date, embryo size, grade and morphology, stallion name and owner name.

14. A 2-quart insulated fluid container with the top removed is filled with liquid nitrogen (Figure 11-2). A cane and goblet (10 mm diameter) is suspended vertically in the liquid nitrogen using forceps. The top of the goblet should be held just above the liquid level so that only liquid nitrogen vapor is within the goblet lumen.

15. Submerge the 0.25 ml straw containing the embryo into liquid nitrogen vapor when the 1-minute countdown ends.

16. Set timer for 1 minute.

17. Plunge the entire cane into liquid nitrogen at the end of the 1-minute period immersing the straw containing the embryo.

18. Transfer into a liquid nitrogen tank for long-term storage.

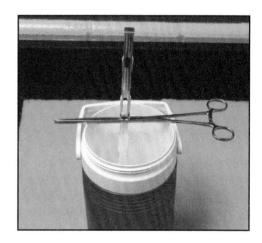

Figure 11-2. Photograph of container of liquid nitrogen with goblet held by forceps.

Warming (Thawing) and Transfer Procedure:

1. The straw containing the correct embryo is identified and removed from long-term storage in the liquid nitrogen tank.

2. The straw is held in room temperature air for 10 seconds.

3. Next, the straw is placed in a room temperature (20 to 22° C) water bath for an additional 10 seconds.

4. The straw is removed from the water bath, wiped dry with a paper towel or Kimwipe™ and then "flicked" like a thermometer 5 to 7 times to mix the galactose dilution solution with the vitrification medium (solution 3) containing the embryo.

5. The straw is then placed in a horizontal position for 6 to 8 minutes. The embryo can be visualized in the straw (and potentially graded) through a microscope (Figure 11-3).

6. The 0.5 ml straw (containing the label information) and plug are removed.

7. The straw is loaded into a sterile sheath and a direct transfer is performed using a Cassou gun.

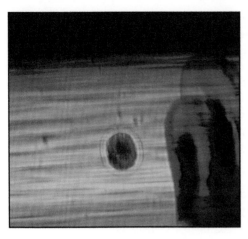

Figure 11-2. Vitrified early blastocyst stage embryo within straw after warming.

Pregnancy Rates after Transfer of Cryopreserved Equine Embryos

In one study pregnancy rates after direct transfer of small vitrified embryos ranged from 62 to 75%. Embryos that were cooled to 5° C and held at that temperature for 12 to 19 hours before vitrification yielded a pregnancy rate of 65% after transfer. The latter study confirmed that embryos could be collected at one location and then cooled and transported to a referral center for cryopreservation.

Pregnancy rates following transfer of a large number of vitrified equine embryos at a large commercial embryo transfer center in the United States compare favorably with pregnancy rates following transfer of fresh or cooled-transported embryos (Table 11-2). In this practice, many of the cryopreserved embryos were collected in the summer and transferred early the following spring.

Table 11-2.
Pregnancy rates following transfer of a total of 4,749 equine embryos at a commercial embryo transfer program (data courtesy of Dr. Jim Bailey and Dr. Ryan Coy, Royal Vista Southwest, Purcell, OK, USA).

Embryo Type	# Embryos Transferred	Pregnancy Rate at Day 11	Pregnancy Rate at Day 25	Live Foal Rate
Fresh	3,060	79.6%	74.6%	68.9%
Cooled	1,479	76.8%	70.2%	64.4%
Frozen	210	70.2%	65.9%	60.4%

Historically, attempts to cryopreserve larger embryos (> 300 μm in diameter) have routinely resulted in pregnancy rates that are quite poor (≤ 20%) after transfer. However, a recent study reported a pregnancy rate of 71% after vitrification of large expanded blastocyst stage embryos following removal of the blastocoele fluid.

Another recent study reported that puncture of the zona pellucida and capsule of embryos 400 to 700 um in diameter followed by removal of the blastocoele fluid and vitrification resulted in satisfactory pregnancy rates after transfer. Additional studies are needed to simplify the procedure for removing blastocoele fluid prior to cryopreservation.

Factors Affecting Pregnancy Rates

Embryo size is a major factor influencing the outcome of cryopreservation. In commercial programs, mares are often palpated once per day to detect ovulation and embryo collection procedures are performed seven or eight days after ovulation. Mean embryo diameters at day seven or eight postovulation are 354.0 ± 13.9 μm and 623.9 ± 72.9 μm, respectively. Numerous studies have reported poor pregnancy rates after transfer for embryos > 300 μm in diameter that have been cryopreserved using slow freezing or vitrification methods.

Other factors that may adversely affect success of cryopreservation of large embryos are the large number of cells that make up an expanded blastocyst, the fluid volume of the blastocoele cavity, and the equine capsule. A day 7 embryo may contain between 272 and 2,117 cells.

The acellular glycoprotein capsule forms beneath the zona pelucida of the early *in vivo* equine embryo. The capsule has been shown to be a barrier to penetration of cryoprotectants into trophoblast cells, the inner cell mass and the blastocoele cavity.

Pregnancy rates are typically lower after transfer of cryopreserved equine embryos than after transfer of fresh or cooled embryos. A pregnancy rate of 65 to 75% would be expected for cryopreserved equine embryos < 300 μm in size.

Suggested Reading

Bruyas J-F. Freezing of Embryos. In: Equine Reproduction, Second Edition. McKinnon AO, Squires EL, Vaala WE, Varner DD (Eds); Wiley-Blackwell, Ames, Iowa 2011; pp. 2287-2290.

Campos-Chillon LF, Suh TK, Barcelo-Fimbres M, Seidel GE Jr., Carnevale EM. Vitrification of early-stage bovine and equine embryos. Theriogenology 2009; 71:349-354.

Carnevale EM. Vitrification of equine embryos. Vet Clin of N Am Equine 2006; 22:831-841.

Carnevale EM, Eldridge-Panuska WD, di Brienza VC. How to collect and vitrify equine embryos for direct transfer. Proceedings Amer Assoc Equine Pract 2004; 50:402-405.

Choi YH, Velez IC, Riera FL, Roldán JE, Hartman DL, Bliss SB, Blanchard TL, Hayden SS, Hinrichs K. Successful cryopreservation of expanded equine blastocysts. Theriogenology 2011; 76:143-152.

Eldridge-Panuska ED, di Brienza VC, Seidel GE Jr., Squires EL, Carnevale EM. Establishment of pregnancies after serial dilution or direct transfer by vitrified equine embryos. Theriogenology 2005; 63:1308-19.

Hinrichs K. Application of assisted reproductive technologies (ART) to clinical practice. Proceedings of the Amer Assoc of Equine Pract 2010; 56:195-206.

Hudson JJ, McCue PM, Carnevale EM, Welsh S, Squires EL. The effects of cooling and vitrification of embryos from mares treated with equine follicle-stimulating hormone on pregnancy rates after nonsurgical transfer. J Equine Vet Sci 2006; 26:51-54.

Squires EL, Carnevale EM, McCue PM, Bruemmer JE. Embryo technologies in the horse. Theriogenology 2003; 59:151-170.

Yamamoto Y, Oguri N, Tsutsumi Y, Hachinohe Y. Experiments in the freezing and storage of equine embryos. J Reprod Fertil, Suppl 1982; 32:399-403.

CHAPTER 12

MANAGEMENT OF RECIPIENTS

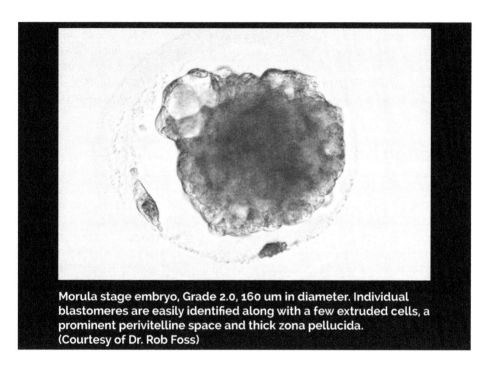

Morula stage embryo, Grade 2.0, 160 um in diameter. Individual blastomeres are easily identified along with a few extruded cells, a prominent perivitelline space and thick zona pellucida.
(Courtesy of Dr. Rob Foss)

Introduction

One of the most important components of any embryo transfer program is the recipient mare. The number of recipients needed for an embryo transfer program is dependent upon the number of donors in the program. If only a single embryo donor is involved a total of two or three recipients should be sufficient to ensure that one recipient mare is synchronized with the donor. Larger embryo transfer facilities will require a greater number of recipient mares, but a lower ratio of recipients to donors.

Acquisition of Recipients

Ideally, recipient mares should be identified and acquired in the fall or early winter prior to the onset of the next breeding season. It would be best to acquire all recipient mares needed for the next season at the same time. This will allow mares to acclimate to their new environment, provide a quarantine period to identify mares with medical issues and prevent exposure of the recipient herd to infectious disease from new mares added to the herd in mid-season.

Selection and Evaluation of Recipients

Recipient mares in large embryo transfer programs are usually maiden or open non-lactating mares between 3 and 12 years of age and weighing between 900 and 1,400 pounds. A recipient mare should be in good physical condition, easy and safe to handle, and have a gentle disposition. Recipient mares should be approximately the same size as the average donor mares. Research has shown that transfer of embryos from a large donor mare into a significantly smaller recipient mare will result in growth restriction of the fetus and birth of a foal that is small for its genetic potential. The size disparity was reported to be still evident at 3 years of age and may persist for life.

A mare may be used as a recipient every-other-year in most ET programs. The recipient mare receives an embryo, becomes pregnant and is sent to the home of the donor mare owner to foal out. The mare foals at home, nurses her foal for 4 to 6 months and is returned to the recipient station in the late summer or fall of the year. She will be put back into the recipient herd and may receive another embryo the following spring. Returned recipients that have done well with previous pregnancies can be used multiple times and may remain in the program well into their teenage years.

Foaling mares can also be used as a recipient. It is advisable to avoid transfer of an embryo after the first postpartum (foal heat) ovulation, but pregnancy rates in subsequent heat cycles should be acceptable.

Barren mares, defined as mares with a history of breeding without a pregnancy, may or may not be good recipient candidates. If a mare cannot become pregnant herself, it is possible that she cannot become pregnant after receiving an embryo.

Initial Evaluation of Potential Recipients

Potential recipient mares should be critically evaluated on arrival and only mares that meet strict criteria are retained as recipients. Maintenance of marginal recipients that are unlikely to receive a client embryo adds to the work load and the cost to maintain the overall program.

A general physical examination should be performed to identify abnormalities of the musculoskeletal system, eyes, oral cavity, mammary gland and other areas. The age of each mare should be estimated during the oral examination. Young mares (< 3 years of age) and aged mares (> 15 years of age) should be identified and not selected as potential recipients. The behavior of each mare should be noted; fractious, dangerous or exceptionally nervous horses are a liability and should not be retained.

A thorough reproductive evaluation should subsequently be performed. The external genitalia should be examined for angle and muscular tone of the vulva. Mares that require a Caslick procedure to prevent aspiration of air may not be ideal recipients. The reproductive tract should be examined by palpation and ultrasound per rectum. The ovaries are examined to determine if both are present and to detect potential abnormalities. Size of follicles, presence of luteal tissue and other significant findings are recorded. The uterus is examined for muscular tone, edema pattern, presence or absence of fluid or air within the uterine lumen, endometrial cysts and other issues. The cervix is also evaluated for tone and morphology.

Uterine culture, cytology and biopsy samples are routinely collected for recipient mares at the initial examination in some embryo transfer programs. In other programs, uterine samples are only collected from mares with uterine fluid identified by transrectal ultrasonography. The goal is to evaluate uterine health and determine if the mare has an infectious or inflammatory condition in the uterus that may adversely affect her ability to become pregnant after transfer or prevent her from carrying a foal to term. Mares with active endometritis should not be used as recipients and it is questionable as to whether or not to retain a mare with endometritis as a potential future recipient mare.

The most common reasons for rejection of a potential recipient mare include musculoskeltal issues (i.e. laminitis, lameness), age, disposition or behavior, uterine abnormalities (i.e. fluid in the uterus, endometritis, endometrial cysts), pregnancy, and ovarian abnormalities (i.e. absence of ovaries, ovarian tumor).

Initial Management of Selected Recipients

Each recipient mare should be identified with a permanent system, such as freeze brands, neck bands, halter tags or microchips. In addition, the physical description of each mare is placed in a permanent medical record.

In most circumstances, the previous deworming and vaccination history of the recipient mare will not be known. Consequently, new recipient mares should be administered an anthelmintic agent and vaccinated against infectious diseases appropriate for specific geographic regions. A blood sample should be collected and tested for equine infectious anemia (Coggins test).

Housing of Recipients

Herds of recipient mares are typically housed in groups of 15 to 25 mares in paddocks or pastures. Mares housed in paddocks are often fed large bales of hay with free access to fresh water and shelter. The paddock system should be designed to allow the herd to be moved as a group to the examination area.

Stress should be minimized in recipient mares. Management procedures to minimize stress would be to avoid overcrowding, avoid moving mares between groups, provide adequate quality, quantity and access to hay or forage, and provide safe shelter.

Seasonal Management

In order to have cycling mares available to receive embryos at the onset of the breeding season, recipients should be maintained under a stimulatory artificial photoperiod beginning on December 1 in North America. Approximately 60 to 70 days of an artificial photoperiod are required to stimulate follicular development and induce ovulation. The most common technique used in recipient mares is outdoor paddock lighting. Timers are used to turn lights on at dusk and turn lights off at 11:00 pm. The goal is to provide a total of 16 hours of light (natural and artificial combined) and allow 8 hours of darkness. The lighting regimen should provide approximately 10 ft-candles of light throughout the paddock.

Gonadotropin releasing hormone (GnRH) or GnRH agonists such as deslorelin acetate have also been used to stimulate follicular development in anestrous or transitional mares (see Formulary in Appendix II). In addition, progesterone therapy may be effective at synchronization of ovulation when administered to mares late in the transition period.

Ultrasound examinations are performed occasionally during deep anestrus (follicles < 20 mm in diameter) and early in the transition period (follicles ≥ 20 mm in diameter). Once the dominant follicle of a transitional mare becomes ≥ 30 mm in diameter, mares are examined every other day. When the dominant follicle is ≥ 35 mm in diameter, the mare may be administered hCG or deslorelin acetate to induce ovulation. Ultrasound examinations are subsequently performed daily to determine the day of ovulation.

If cycling recipients are not available early in the breeding season, noncycling or ovariectomized mares administered gonadal steroids can be used as recipients. A noncycling mare can be administered 5 to 10 mg of estradiol-17β (E_2) intramuscularly once daily for 2 to 4 days when the donor mare is in estrus and then administered altrenogest or progesterone beginning one or two days after ovulation of the donor mare. Since the donor mare is usually flushed 7 or 8 days after ovulation, the noncycling mare would have received progesterone for 5 to 7 days before receiving an embryo.

Unfortunately, pregnancy rates are usually slightly lower following transfer of an embryo into a hormone-treated noncycling or ovariectomized mare than following transfer into a synchronized cycling mare.

Synchronization of Recipients and Donors

Synchronization of an individual donor and a single recipient mare may be requested by an owner. If the owner is providing the recipient(s), it is recommended that 2 to 3 recipients be synchronized along with the donor in order that at least one recipient mare ovulates during the critical time window. Ideally, the recipient mare would have ovulated 1-2 days after the donor mare.

Synchronization of estrus and ovulation can be accomplished by one of three techniques: 1) administration of two doses of prostaglandins 14 days apart, 2) administration of progesterone or a synthetic progestin once daily for 10 days plus a single dose of prostaglandins on the last day of progestin therapy, and 3) administration of progesterone or progestin for 14-15 days. The easiest technique is administration of two doses of prostaglandins 14 days apart. The tightest degree of synchrony is achieved by daily administration progesterone plus estradiol for 10 days followed by prostaglandin administration. Exogenous progesterone and estradiol will suppress both pituitary LH and FSH secretion, resulting in an overall suppression of ovarian follicular development. Follicular growth will resume when "P+E" therapy is discontinued. It may be beneficial to stagger the onset of therapy in donors and recipients to increase the probability that the recipient mare(s) will ovulate slightly after the donor mare.

Once the donor and recipient(s) are in estrus, appropriate synchronization of ovulation can be obtained by administration of either hCG or deslorelin. The recipient mare is usually administered hCG or deslorelin the day ovulation has been confirmed in the donor mare. Consequently, ovulation in the recipient should occur 1-2 days after the donor mare.

Estrous synchronization is not typically required in large embryo transfer programs as there are usually enough mares that ovulate spontaneously on any given day to accommodate the embryos collected. However, it may be necessary to modulate the herd ovulation pattern by strategic use of prostaglandins to avoid large time periods without ovulations. Recipient mares that do not receive an embryo are usually administered prostaglandins 9 or 10 days after ovulation to cause luteolysis and an early return to estrus.

On a rare occasion an embryo has been transferred back into the original donor mare successfully when two embryos were collected and only one recipient was available.

Routine Examination of Recipient Mares

Recipient mares are examined on the day of prostaglandin administration. The reasons for an ultrasound examination prior to prostaglandin administration are to 1) confirm the identity of the mare, 2) confirm that the mare is not pregnant, 3) confirm the presence of a corpus luteum, and 4) determine the size of the largest follicle, which will help predict the interval to subsequent ovulation. In general, the interval to ovulation is longer in mares with small follicles at the time of prostaglandin administration (Table 12-1).

Table 12-1.
Interval from prostaglandin administration to spontaneous ovulation based on follicle diameter at the time of treatment.

Follicle Diameter at PGF	Interval to Ovulation (days)
10 mm	9 to 12 days
20 mm	8 to 11 days
25 mm	6 to 10 days
30 mm	5 to 9 days
≥ 35 mm	*Possible outcomes* • May ovulate dominant follicle within 1-2 days • May ovulate dominant follicle 3 or more days after PGF • May regress the dominant follicle and develop another follicle that ovulates 10 to 12 days after PGF

Timing of subsequent examinations is dependent on size of the largest follicle at the time of prostaglandin administration. In most instances, a mare will be examined 4 days after prostaglandin administration. Mares are examined every 2-3 days until a dominant follicle is ≥ 35 mm in diameter, after which the mare is examined once daily to determine the day of ovulation.

All recipients are examined 5 days after ovulation to determine if they qualify to receive an embryo on that cycle. Mares that are graded as "acceptable" on this examination are available for use as recipients for the next 3-4 days. Pregnancy rates are generally higher for recipients that are graded as "acceptable" on the "5-day Check" versus mares that are graded as "marginally acceptable" or "unacceptable".

A recipient mare may be selected to receive a specific embryo based on the following criteria:
• Day of ovulation relative to the donor mare
• Day of ovulation relative to size and developmental stage of the embryo
• Quality of estrous cycle
• Presence and quality of the corpus luteum
• Progesterone level (optional)
• Tone of the uterus
• Tone of the cervix
• Absence of uterine edema
• Size of the recipient relative to size of the donor mare
• General physical health
• Behavioral characteristics
• Absence of reproductive abnormalities, medical issues or behavioral concerns

Many factors can be used to disqualify or decrease the likelihood of using a certain recipient mare as a candidate for receiving an embryo. These factors include:
• Poor quality cycle
• Ovulation within 2 days after receiving prostaglandins
• Ovulation of an abnormally small follicle

- Failure of ovulation or development of a hemorrhagic anovulatory follicle
- Absence of uterine edema during the cycle
- Presence of echogenic fluid within the uterine lumen during estrus
- Presence of fluid within the uterine lumen during diestrus
- Presence of a significant medical condition or behavioral issue
- Failure to form a corpus luteum after ovulation
- Low progesterone (optional)
- Small corpus luteum
- Presence of uterine edema during diestrus
- Poor tone in the uterus or cervix during diestrus

Equine embryos are collected on either day 6, 7, 8 or 9 after ovulation of the donor mare. Embryos are usually transferred into a recipient mare that ovulated during a window that may range from one day prior to the donor mare (+1 synchrony) to 3 days after ovulation of the donor mare (-3 synchrony). It is a common opinion that pregnancy rates are highest if the embryo is transferred into a recipient that ovulated 1 or 2 days after the donor (Table 12-2). Pregnancy rates are significantly lower if an embryo is transferred into a recipient mare that ovulated 2 or more days prior to the donor mare. Pregnancies can be obtained from embryos transferred into a recipient that ovulated 4 or 5 days after the donor mare. However, in commercial programs it may be necessary to utilize recipients that ovulated the same day as the donor (0 synchrony) or one day prior to the donor (+1) and save recipients that have recently ovulated for embryos to be collected in the near future. It is recommended that one always looks ahead at upcoming flushes in the next 2 to 3 days before making a final decision on recipients.

Ideally several recipient mares would be available to choose from for each embryo recovered. Consequently the best recipient mare could be selected to match the donor mare, the ovulation day and the developmental stage of the embryo.

Recipient mares may receive 2 or maximally 3 embryos in a given year. If they do not become pregnant or if they lose a pregnancy after 2 or 3 opportunities, they are generally culled from the recipient herd.

Table 12-2.
Synchrony between donor mare that ovulated 7 days prior to embryo collection and potential recipient mares that ovulated between 2 days before to 3 days after the donor mare. Comments regarding order of selection of the recipient are also presented.

Donor Flush Day	Recipient Ovulation Day	Synchrony	Selection Comments
	d 9	+2	Not acceptable
	d 8	+1	Use if needed
Day 7	d 7	0	3rd Choice
	d 6	-1	1st Choice
	d 5	-2	2nd Choice
	d 4	-3	Use if needed

Recommended Reading

Allen WR, Wilsher S, Tiplady C, Butterfield RM. The influence of maternal size on pre- and postnatal growth in the horse: III Postnatal growth. Reproduction 2004;127:67-77.

Lagneaux D, Palmer E. Are pony and larger mares similar as recipients for non-surgical transfer of Day 7 embryos? Equine Vet J 1989;Suppl 8:64-67.

McCue PM, Gee EK, Magee C, Woods GL, Squires EL. 2007, Hormones and other medical therapies in embryo transfer recipient mares. Embryo Transfer Proceedings, Society for Theriogenology August 7-11, Monterey, California. p. 27-35.

Riera F. General techniques and organization of large commercial embryo transfer programs. Clinical Theriogenology 2011;3:318-324.

Squires EL, Seidel Jr GE. Collection and transfer of equine embryos. Colorado State University Animal Reproduction and Biotechnology Laboratory Bulletin No. 8, 1995; 64 pp.

CHAPTER 13

TRANSFER OF EQUINE EMBRYOS

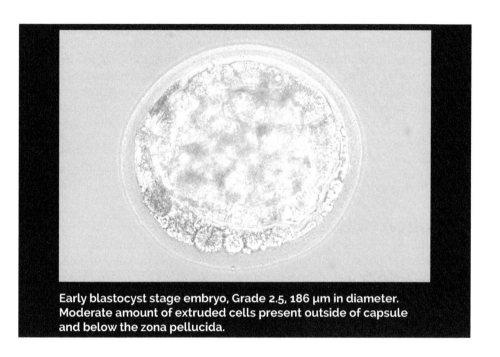

Early blastocyst stage embryo, Grade 2.5, 186 μm in diameter. Moderate amount of extruded cells present outside of capsule and below the zona pellucida.

Introduction

Transfer of an embryo into a recipient mare is where the art and science of equine embryo transfer merge. Research studies and years of anecdotal clinical evidence have provided a wealth of information on handling of embryos, evaluation of embryos, selection of the optimal recipient for a given embryo, and transfer of an embryo into the uterus of a recipient mare. In addition, specialized equipment and disposable supplies have been designed for the handling and transfer of equine embryos.

Historically, many equine embryos were transferred surgically into the uterus of a recipient. A combination of increased knowledge of equine reproductive physiology, improvement in embryo transfer equipment and adjustments in clinical techniques have led to improved pregnancy rates following nonsurgical transfer. Currently routine equine embryo transfers are performed using a nonsurgical, trans-cervical procedure. The only exception is that some cleavage-stage or other early developmental stage equine embryos produced by intra-cytoplasmic sperm injection **(ICSI)** or other *in vitro* techniques may require surgical transfer into the oviduct of a recipient mare.

Equine embryos are expensive and sometimes difficult to obtain. Sufficient care should be taken during recipient selection and transfer of the embryo to optimize success.

Selection of the Recipient Mare

The reproductive cycle of the recipient mares should be closely monitored by palpation and ultrasonography per rectum. The goal is to evaluate ovarian follicular development, endometrial edema pattern, follicle size at ovulation, determine the day of ovulation and number of ovulations, monitor development of the corpus luteum, and detect reproductive abnormalities. Recipient mares suspected of having any significant reproductive pathology should be evaluated appropriately and should not receive an embryo until the problem is identified and resolved.

Initial selection of a recipient candidate is based on ovulation dates and synchronization with the donor. However, if a small embryo (i.e. < 200 μm diameter) of an early developmental stage (i.e. morula or early blastocyst) is collected from a mare that ovulated 8 days previously, it may be advantageous to select a recipient mare that lines up more with the developmental stage of the embryo rather than the ovulation date of the donor. Consequently, one might select a recipient mare that ovulated 5 days previously (-3 synchrony) rather than a mare that ovulated 8 or 9 days previously (i.e. a 0 or +1 synchrony).

Quality of the estrous cycle leading to ovulation should be taken into consideration when selecting the specific recipient for a given embryo. Rate of follicular growth, interval from prostaglandin administration to ovulation, diameter of the dominant follicle at ovulation, pattern of uterine edema, presence or absence of free fluid within the uterine lumen during estrus, and confirmation of an actual ovulation are all important factors in recipient selection. In some instances, it is as much about eliminating poor recipient candidates as it is about identifying a good recipient candidate.

In a vast majority of mares, a morphologically normal corpus luteum will be present when the recipient mare is examined 5 days after ovulation (i.e. "5-Day Check"). However, a small corpus luteum or no visible corpus luteum may be noted in a low percentage of mares on the "5-Day Check". Plasma progesterone levels have been determined to be significantly higher in mares that qualified as potential recipients (10.0 ± 4.2 ng/ml) as compared to mares that failed to qualify (6.5 ± 4.3 ng/ml) based on palpation and ultrasound examination of the ovaries, uterus and cervix.

An elevated progesterone level is usually associated with an absence of uterine edema and the presence of good muscular tone in the uterus and cervix. Conversely, the presence of uterine edema and poor tone of the uterus or cervix is associated with a low concentration of endogenous progesterone and often disqualify a mare as a recipient prospect for that cycle. Evaluation of progesterone levels is not a routine criterion for selection of a recipient mare due to expense and lack of a rapid, quantitative progesterone assay for the horse.

Another criterion for selection of the optimal recipient mare for a specific embryo is related to the size of the donor mare versus the size of the recipient mare and the physical health and temperament of the recipient mare. Ideally, one would select a recipient mare that is of similar size to the donor mare, is in good physical health and has a gentle disposition.

A final evaluation of the chosen recipient mare is usually performed immediately prior to receiving an embryo. It is optimal to have more than one recipient candidate available in case one is determined to be unsatisfactory.

Preparation of the Recipient Mare for Transfer
Sedation
Recipient mares are often sedated 5 to 10 minutes prior to the transfer procedure. The most common medications administered are acepromazine maleate (10 to 20 mg, i.v.), xylazine hydrochloride (150 to 200 mg, i.v.) or detomidine hydrochloride (5 to 7.5 mg, i.v.). Acepromazine is an α_1-adrenergic receptor antagonist while xylazine and detomidine are both α_2-adrenergic receptor agonists. Administration of acepromazine during diestrus may cause suppression of myometrial activity for 90 minutes and clinically result in decreased uterine tone, moderate relaxation of the cervix and mild relaxation of the vulva.

Administration of xylazine or detomidine during diestrus will increase myometrial activity for 30 minutes and 60 minutes, respectively and clinically result in an increase in uterine tone with no perceptible changes in the cervix or vulva. There is no clear consensus as to which sedation medication is more advantageous and personal preference of the transfer technician generally dictates which drug, if any, is used.

Non-Steroidal Anti-Inflammatory Medications
Cervical manipulation during nonsurgical embryo transfer may be associated with oxytocin and/or prostaglandin release which may subsequently cause an alteration

of luteal function. Consequently, it has become standard practice to administer a prostaglandin synthesis inhibitor prior to nonsurgical embryo transfer in horses, the most common of which is flunixin meglumine. Flunixin meglumine inhibits the enzymes COX-1 and COX-2 which convert free arachadonic acid to prostaglandin G_2 and prostaglandin H_2, respectively, and is therefore considered to be a non-specific inhibitor of prostaglandin synthesis.

Meclofenamic acid is another non-steroidal anti-inflammatory drug **(NSAID)** which prevents production of prostaglandins through an inhibition of prostaglandin H synthase. It has been reported that administration of meclofenamic acid to recipient mares that ovulated 2 or more days prior to the donor mare (i.e. +2 or more asynchronous recipient mares) may allow for successful establishment of pregnancies after transfer.

Corticosteroids
Corticosteroids are sometimes administered prior to nonsurgical embryo transfer in an attempt to suppress inflammation and prostaglandin release that may occur secondary to cervical-uterine manipulation. However, controlled studies have not been reported.

Antibiotics
Systemic antibiotics may be administered to recipient mares prior to and following transfer of an embryo in an attempt to decrease the probability of embryonic loss secondary to bacterial contamination. Antibiotics are not routinely administered at most embryo transfer centers. However, systemic antibiotics may be beneficial if a recipient is transferred an embryo covered with debris, if the flush effluent contained significant debris or if the embryo was recovered from a mare with a history of bacterial endometritis.

Tocolytic Agents
Terbutaline sulfate, clenbuterol, and isoxsuprine hydrochloride all have the capability of reducing uterine contractions when administered to mares. Terbutaline (15 mg) has been used in an equine embryo transfer program to decrease uterine contractions stimulated by cervical or uterine manipulations and prevent the active expulsion of the transferred embryo. The need for a tocolytic agent administered prior to transcervical equine embryo transfer is not clear. A majority of commercial embryo transfer centers do not use tocolytic agents prior to transfer and report acceptable pregnancy rates.

Anticholinergic agents
The anticholinergic drug N-butylscopolammonium bromide (Buscopan™ Injectable Solution, Boehringer Ingelheim Vetmedica, Inc.) administered at a dose of 0.04 to 0.08 mg/kg (i.e. a total dose of 20 to 40 mg in a 500 kg mare) has been reported to induce relaxation of the rectal musculature and may therefore reduce the potential risk of injury to the rectum during reproductive procedures such as nonsurgical embryo transfer that may involve palpation per rectum.

The drug has a rapid onset of activity (< 1 minute) after intravenous administration and a 15 to 25 minute duration of action. Propantheline bromide (PRO-BANTHINE®) is a synthetic quaternary ammonium anticholinergic agent which inhibits gastro-intestinal motility and spasm. It may also be used to induce rectal relaxation as an aid to non-surgical embryo transfer.

Transfer Technique

The tail of the recipient is wrapped and held away from the perineal area. The perineum is washed with warm water and a non-residual soap two or three consecutive times until clean. The area is subsequently rinsed with a copious volume of fresh water and dried with paper towels. The vestibule should be swabbed with a pledget of moist cotton or paper towels to remove any organic debris that may contaminate the uterus of the recipient mare during transfer.

There are many sources of equipment and supplies for transfer of equine embryos (Appendix 1). Embryos less than 1,000 µm in diameter are often transferred using a 0.25ml straw, disposable sterile sheath and stainless steel Cassou gun (IMV International Corp, Minneapolis, MN). The straw is connected to a 1.0 or 3.0 ml syringe using a ureteral catheter connector. A column of holding medium is drawn up into the straw (approximately 50 % of the straw). A small air gap is added prior to another small column of fluid followed by a second air gap. The embryo is subsequently drawn up into the straw within a small column of fluid. Straw filling is completed with two more small fluid columns and air gaps. It is important to make sure the first (larger) column of fluid makes contact with the plug of the straw. This will seal the straw and prevent the fluid and embryo from leaking out of the straw. Ultimately the embryo is confined to the center of the straw, with one or two air gaps on either side (Figure 13-1). The air gaps are important to confine the embryo to the center of the straw and to help expel the embryo from the straw at transfer. The straw is loaded into the disposable sheath which is then attached to the Cassou gun.

Embryos greater than 1,000 µm in diameter are commonly transferred using a standard artificial insemination pipette, which is attached to a 1.0 or 3.0 ml syringe. A small volume of holding medium is drawn up into the pipette, followed by a small air

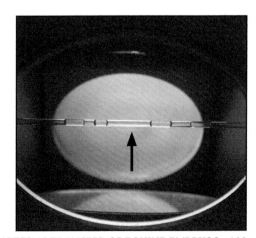

Figure 13-1. Embryo (arrow) confined between two air gaps within a 0.25 ml straw.

gap. The embryo is then aspirated into the pipette within a small volume of fluid. This is followed by another air gap and a final small volume of fluid. Ultimately the embryo is contained within a small column of fluid (total volume of approximately 1.0 ml) surrounded by one air gap on either side.

With either the Cassou gun system or the pipette system, it is recommended that a sterile outer chemise be used to protect the transfer gun or pipette from contamination with bacteria from the vulva, vestibule or vagina.

The tip of the transfer instrument, within the protective chemise, is held within a hand covered by a sterile obstetrical sleeve to which a small volume of sterile lubricant has been applied (Figure 13-2). The hand and instrument are passed into the caudal reproductive tract and directed forward to the cranial portion of the vaginal vault. An important aspect of transcervical embryo transfer is to minimize manipulation of the cervix. The cervix of a recipient mare in diestrus should be tightly closed. Insertion of a finger into the cervix in order to guide the transfer instrument into the uterus should be avoided, as it may cause prostaglandin release or may transfer bacterial organisms into the cervix or uterus. It has been estimated that the simple act of inserting a finger into the cervix will reduce transfer success rate (i.e. decrease pregnancy rate in recipient mares) by 10 to 15 % or more. Instead, one can encircle the external portion of the cervix with an index finger and thumb and use the palm of the hand to direct the tip of the transfer instrument into the external cervical os. The protective chemise should be pulled caudally using the hand outside the mare to allow the tip of the transfer instrument (Cassou gun or pipette) to penetrate the cranial aspect of the chemise at the entrance to the external cervical os.

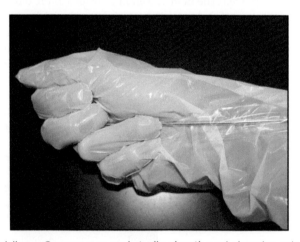

Figure 13-2. Holding a Cassou gun and sterile sheath and chemise prior to transfer.

The transfer instrument can be gently manipulated from the outside to maneuver the tip of the instrument within the cervical lumen and with a gentle steady forward motion facilitate passage of the instrument into the uterine body. The embryo may be deposited into the uterine body without any additional manipulations. Alternatively, the transfer technician can gently guide the instrument into one uterine horn via manipulation per rectum. The embryo should be gently deposited within the center of the uterine lumen as the transfer instrument is slowly withdrawn. Consistent success is aided by attention to detail and a delicate transfer technique.

Alternatively, a technique has been described for transcervical transfer using a special instrument (Wilsher forceps) designed to grasp the ventral external cervical os and retract it caudally to straighten the cervix and consequently facilitate passage of the Cassou gun or pipette through the cervical canal.

Examination of the Transfer Instrument after Transfer

Observations from ET personnel using the Cassou gun system indicate that embryos occasionally become caught in the side ejecting stainless steel tip of the disposable sheath. Consequently, it is recommended that the tip of the sheath be rinsed after transfer and the rinse fluid examined under a microscope. A retrospective study at Colorado State University revealed that 5 of 820 transfer procedures (0.6%) were associated with an embryo that failed to be discharged from the tip of the transfer gun. In each case, the embryo was loaded into a new straw and sterile sheath and immediately retransferred into the same recipient mare. Pregnancies were obtained in 3 of the 5 recipient mares after "re-transfer".

Failure to examine the sheath after transfer may result in the inadvertent loss of an embryo. It should not be presumed that an embryo has been safely transferred into a recipient until the tip of the transfer gun has been examined.

Management of the Recipient Mare after Transfer

Minimizing stress in the recipient mare after transfer is important to optimize pregnancy rates. Consequently, it may be beneficial to keep the recipient mare in her original herd after transfer as opposed to moving her immediately to a different herd of post-transfer mares. Anecdotal evidence suggests that social stress may adversely affect pregnancy rates in recipient mares.

It is probable that most embryo transfer recipient mares do not need supplemental progesterone. However, administration of exogenous progesterone or progestins to recipient mares following embryo transfer is routinely performed at some embryo transfer facilities and used sparingly or not at all at other facilities. The decision whether or not to supplement with progesterone is based on clinical experience, value of the embryo, and the perceived risk that luteal insufficiency may adversely affect embryonic survival in a given mare. It has been documented that the nonsurgical transcervical procedure is occasionally associated with complete luteolysis (Figure 13-3).

If progesterone supplementation is provided, recipient mares may receive either altrenogest (0.044 mg/kg; orally, once daily), progesterone-in-oil (200 mg, intra muscularly, once daily), or a long-acting progesterone (1,500 mg, intramuscularly, once every 7 days). Altrenogest is the only progestin approved for use in the horse.

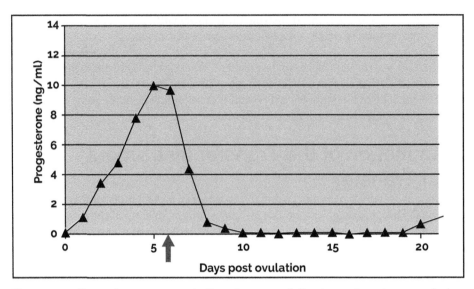

Figure 13-3. Progesterone concentrations in a mare following a sham transcervical transfer procedure. Note that progesterone levels declined to < 1.0 ng/ml within 24 hours after the procedure.

Advantages of altrenogest therapy are: 1) administration orally or in grain is easy to administer and readily accepted by the mare, 2) endogenous progesterone can still be measured, as the antibody used in progesterone assays will not detect altrenogest, and 3) a non-pregnant recipient will begin to cycle back immediately after daily oral altrenogest therapy is discontinued.

Progesterone-in-oil has a short half-life and requires daily intramuscular administration, which may occasionally be associated with inflammation at the injection sites and resentment by the mare. Long-acting progesterone has the advantage of less frequent administration, but may also be associated with inflammation at the injection site(s). In addition, there may be a delay in return to estrus for non-pregnant recipient mares after discontinuation of long-acting progesterone therapy.

If supplemental progesterone therapy is used in intact, cycling recipient mares, it is often initiated at the time the embryo is transferred. If the recipient mare is not pregnant on a day 16 (embryo age) ultrasound examination, supplementation is discontinued and the mare is allowed to return to estrus. Prostaglandins may be administered when progesterone therapy is discontinued in the non-pregnant recipient.

If the recipient mare is pregnant and on progesterone supplementation, it is recommended that therapy be continued beyond the time of maternal recognition of pregnancy (day 12 to 16 post ovulation). The uterus of some pregnant recipient mares may not recognize that an embryo is present. This may be especially true for mares that received a small embryo of an early developmental stage (i.e. a morula or early blastocyst). Consequently, the endometrium of the pregnant recipient mare may release prostaglandins which causes luteolysis and eliminates endogenous progesterone support.

Progesterone supplementation may be discontinued at any time provided that endogenous levels are measured and determined to be sufficient to maintain pregnancy (Table 13-1). Endogenous progesterone levels may be measured if the mare is supplemented with altrenogest, as the antibody in most progesterone assays will not "detect" or cross react with this synthetic progestin. In contrast, an accurate assessment of endogenous progesterone is not possible in mares supplemented with natural progesterone.

Table 13-1.
Options for discontinuation of progesterone or progestin therapy in a pregnant recipient mare.

Day	Data Required	Comments
Day 16 to 120	Endogenous P_4 Level	Progesterone level of > 4.0 ng/ml should be adequate to maintain pregnancy
Day 45 to 70	Ultrasound detection of secondary CLs	Secondary corpora lutea formation is associated with increased progesterone production, which should be sufficient to maintain pregnancy
Day 120+	Ultrasound confirmation of pregnancy	The placenta should be producing sufficient progestins to maintain pregnancy
Full term	Recipient is close to her calculated due date	It is rarely required or recommended that a recipient mare be maintained on supplemental progesterone throughout the entire length of gestation. However, if warranted, the recipient may be administered supplemental progesterone until the day she foals

Progesterone therapy in a recipient mare may be discontinued between 45 to 70 days of pregnancy if an ultrasound examination confirms the presence of secondary corpora lutea (Figure 13-4). Alternatively, progesterone or progestin therapy may be discontinued at approximately 120 days of gestation without testing to determine concentrations of endogenous progesterone. The placenta produces sufficient progesterone and other progestins by day 90 to maintain the pregnancy.

Another approach to progesterone supplementation is to provide progesterone to an intact cycling recipient mare only if: 1) the uterine and cervical tone is less than that considered adequate or the size or appearance of the corpus luteum prior to transfer is considered abnormal, 2) the corpus luteum appears to be small or regressing or a small amount of uterine edema is present on a 14 to 16 day ultrasound examination, and/or 3) serum progesterone levels are < 4.0 ng/ml either prior to transfer or after the initial pregnancy examination (Figures 13-5 & 13-6). Blood samples may be collected periodically from the recipient mares to confirm if endogenous progesterone levels are high enough to maintain the pregnancy. Altrenogest treatment may be discontinued at owner request if progesterone levels are > 4.0 ng/ml.

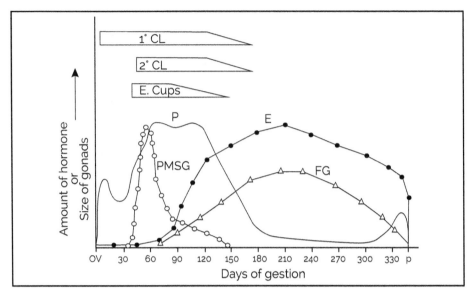

Figure 13-4. Endocrinology of pregnancy. Note the rise in progesterone *(P)* that coincides with formation of secondary corpora lutea *(2° CL)*. PMSG, pregnant mare serum gonadotropin, currently termed equine chorionic gonadotropin *(eCG)*, 1° CL, primary corpus luteum; E. Cups, endometrial cups; E, estrogens; FG, fetal gonads; OV, ovulation; p, parturition. (From Squires EL. Endocrinology of pregnancy. In: Equine Reproduction. AO McKinnon and JL Voss Editors, Williams & Wilkins, Baltimore; 1993, pp. 495-500).

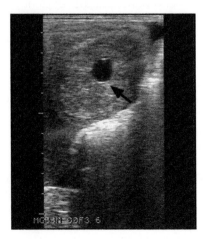
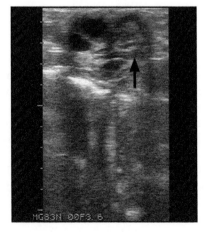

Figure 13-5. Ultrasound photos of a mare on day 14 with an embryonic vesicle (arrow) within the uterus (left photo) and a regressing corpus luteum (arrow) within the ovary (right photo). Progesterone level was 2.4 ng/ml.

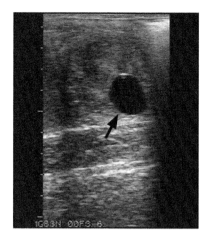 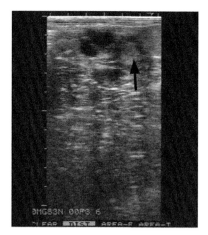

Figure 13-6. Ultrasound photos of the same mare at day 16, showing the embryonic vesicle (arrow) within the uterus (left photo) and a remnant of luteal tissue (arrow) within the ovary (right photo). Progesterone level was 0.7 ng/ml. The recipient mare remained pregnant due to daily altrenogest therapy.

Suggested Reading

Foss R, Wirth N, Schiltz P, Jones J. Nonsurgical embryo transfer in a private practice (1998). Proceedings of the 45th Annual Convention of the American Association of Equine Pract 1999; 45:210-212.

McCue PM, Gee EK, Magee C, Woods GL, Squires EL. 2007, Hormones and other medical therapies in embryo transfer recipient mares. Embryo Transfer Proceedings, Society for Theriogenology August 7-11, Monterey, California. p. 27-35.

McCue, PM, Vanderwall DK, Keith SL and Squires EL. 1999, Equine embryo transfer: influence of endogenous progesterone concentration in recipients on pregnancy outcome. Theriogenology 51: 267.

Wilsher S, Kölling M, Allen WR. Meclofenamic acid extends donor-recipient asynchrony in equine embryo transfer. Equine Vet Journal 2006; 38:428-432.

CHAPTER 14

PREGNANCY EXAMINATION AFTER TRANSFER

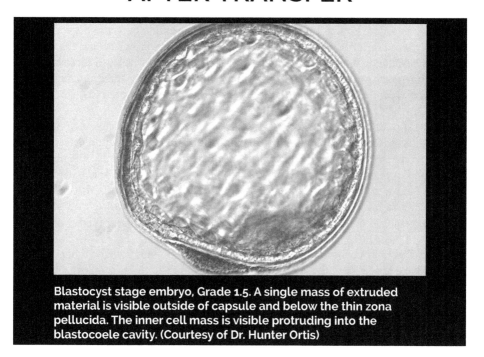

Blastocyst stage embryo, Grade 1.5. A single mass of extruded material is visible outside of capsule and below the thin zona pellucida. The inner cell mass is visible protruding into the blastocoele cavity. (Courtesy of Dr. Hunter Ortis)

Introduction

An initial ultrasound pregnancy examination of the recipient mare is usually performed 4 to 7 days after transfer, which usually corresponds to an embryo age of 11 to 14 days. The advantage of an early pregnancy examination (i.e. 4 days after transfer) is that the donor mare can be managed appropriately as she is coming back into heat based on the presence or absence of a pregnancy in the recipient mare.

Ultrasound Pregnancy Examinations

A thorough, systematic approach to ultrasonographic pregnancy diagnosis is imperative in order to correctly diagnose pregnancy status and detect twins which can (rarely) occur after transfer of a single embryo. It is recommended that the entire uterus be scanned in one continuous motion in order to avoid missing a section of the uterus. The most common locations for a single embryo or a twin embryo to be missed are the caudal uterine body adjacent to the cervix and the tip of a uterine horn.

The uterus should be examined for the presence of an embryonic vesicle and potential abnormalities including uterine edema, free fluid in the uterus, and endometrial cysts. The embryonic vesicle may be first visible by ultrasound on day 10 or 11. The ultrasonographic appearance of the equine embryo changes from a round shape (day 10 to 16) to a more triangular shape on day 17 to 21. Growth rate of the vesicle plateaus between 17 and 24 days, after which growth resumes at a slightly slower rate. The developing embryonic vesicle may have a somewhat irregular shape from day 25 to 35.

An embryo proper may become visible 20 to 23 days after ovulation and a heart-beat can usually be observed within the embryo proper by day 24 to 25. A follow-up examination with ultrasonography is generally recommended between 25 and 35 days of pregnancy to confirm that the pregnancy is still viable.

Ultrasonographic images of early equine pregnancies are presented in Figures 14-1 to 14-4.

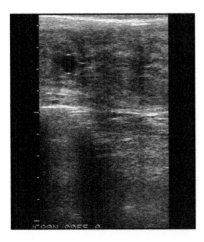

Figure 14-1. Ultrasound image of a 12 day pregnancy.

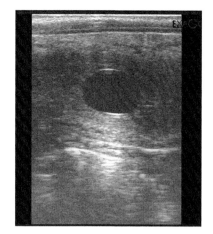

Figure 14-2. Ultrasound image of a 16 day pregnancy.

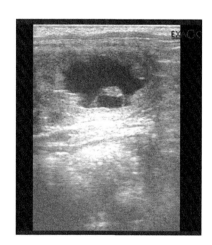

Figure 14-3. Ultrasound image of a 25 day pregnancy.

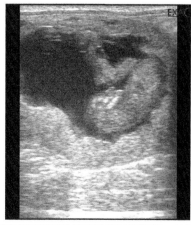

Figure 14-4. Ultrasound image of a 50 day pregnancy.

Pregnancy Detection

A retrospective study was performed on data from 584 recipient mares that were confirmed to be pregnant at a day 16 ultrasound examination. All donor mares were flushed 7 days after ovulation. An initial pregnancy exam was performed 4 days after transfer (day 11 embryo age) and subsequent examinations were performed at day 12, 14 and 16. An embryonic vesicle was first detected in 76.4 % of the mares on the day 11 examination. A positive pregnancy diagnosis was obtained during 92.9% of ultrasound examinations performed on day 12 and 98.9% of examinations performed at day 14. The mean diameter of embryos at the time of transfer that resulted in a positive pregnancy examination at day 11 (469.6 ± 13.0 μm) was greater (p<0.05) than the diameter of embryos that were not associated with a positive pregnancy examination at day 11 (300.0 ± 20.8 μm), but the recipient mare was subsequently determined to be pregnant.

In summary, ultrasound examination at day 11 is often able to confirm the presence of an embryonic vesicle if a large embryo was initially transferred. However, pregnancy may not be initially detected at day 11 in mares that receive a small embryo, but the embryo may become visible on ultrasound on day 12, 14 or 16 (embryo age). The clinical significance is that donor mares flushed at day 7 and administered prostaglandins after the flush are usually back in heat 4 to 6 days after the collection procedure and ready to be rebred by 7 to 9 days after the flush. An early accurate pregnancy diagnosis is critical to facilitate subsequent reproductive management of the donor mare.

Embryonic Development

Equine embryos grow an average of 3 to 5 mm per day from day 11 to day 16 of pregnancy (Table 14-1). Failure to grow, reduced growth rate, or failure to advance in developmental stage may be associated with eventual embryo loss.

Table 14-1.
Diameter of the embryonic vesicle in pregnant recipient mares on days 11 to 16 (embryo age).

Day of Pregnancy	Embryonic Vesicle Diameter (mm)
11	5.5 ± 0.1
12	8.5 ± 0.1
14	14.9 ± 0.2
16	23.5 ± 0.2

Ovarian Examination

The ovaries should be evaluated during all pregnancy examinations for the presence and physical characteristics of the corpus luteum. The primary corpus luteum should be visible and morphologically normal in a pregnant recipient mare up to day 45. Supplementary corpora lutea may be identified in pregnant mares after 45 to 60 days of gestation (Figure 14-5). Multiple supplementary CL's may be present on each ovary and the size of the ovary is subsequently increased. It should be noted that not every pregnant mare develops supplementary corpora lutea. Observation of supplementary CL's may be important for management decisions as to whether or not to continue administration of exogenous progesterone or progestins.

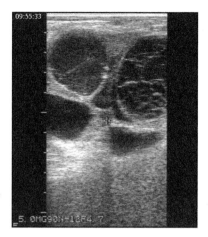

Figure 14-5. Ultrasonographic image of multiple supplementary corpora lutea in a pregnant mare.

Progesterone Evaluation

Progesterone measurement is valuable in determining if a pregnant mare is producing sufficient progesterone to maintain her pregnancy. Generally, a serum concentration of ≥ 4 ng/ml is considered adequate to maintain pregnancy when measured during the first 2 to 3 months of gestation when the ovary is the primary source of progesterone. Progesterone levels may rise substantially by day 60 in mares that form supplementary corpora lutea.

Interpretation of progesterone levels in samples collected after day 100 are more complicated. The equine placenta produces a variety of progestin compounds that are often either not detected in a standard progesterone assay or have limited cross reactivity in the assay. Progesterone assays typically utilize an antibody specific for progesterone (P_4), with some potential cross-reactivity with other natural progestagens. Evaluation of a blood sample collected during the second half of pregnancy may reveal a "progesterone" level between 2.5 and 4.0 ng/ml, which would be low for a mare in early pregnancy. However, other progestogens are being produced which help with maintenance of pregnancy (Figure 14-6). Therefore, interpretation of progesterone values must be based on the stage of pregnancy and used cautiously after day 100.

Abnormalities Detected During a Pregnancy Examination

Abnormalities detected during ultrasound pregnancy examinations include uterine edema, presence of a very small corpus luteum, absence of a corpus luteum, presence of one or more endometrial cysts, fluid in the uterine lumen, twins, absence of a pregnancy, presence of a dead embryo or fetus, and presence of an empty trophoblastic vesicle.

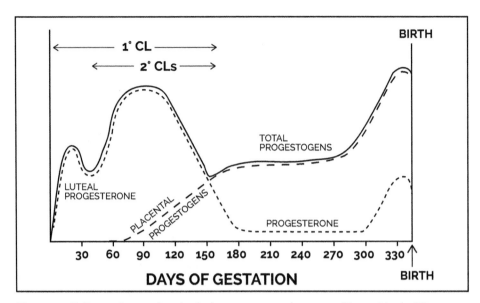

Figure 14-6. Progesterone levels during pregnancy in mares. (From: Neely DP. Gestation. In: Equine Reproduction. Neely DP, Liu IKM, Hillman RB, Editors, Veterinary Learning Systems Co., Inc. 1983, pp. 58-70).

Edema

Uterine or endometrial edema is usually associated with an elevated estradiol level and a low progesterone level. Edema should not be present in a pregnant mare. Detection of endometrial edema in a pregnant mare (Figure 14-7) suggests low endogenous progesterone levels. As a consequence, progesterone support should be instituted immediately. In most instances progesterone or progestin supplementation can rescue the pregnancy even in the absence of significant endogenous progesterone production.

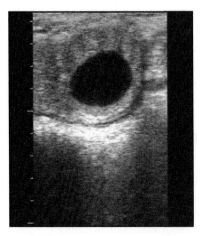

Figure 14-7. Edema in a pregnant mare. Note the radiating pattern within the endometrium.

Small Corpus Luteum

Detection of a small corpus luteum (Figure 14-8) or absence of the corpus luteum on days 11 to 16 in a pregnant mare suggests failure of maternal recognition of pregnancy and a lack of progesterone support. Progesterone supplementation should be instituted immediately. A blood sample may be collected for confirmation of progesterone levels, if desired. It should be noted that evaluation of a single blood sample prior to day 16 may not be indicative of true luteal function as levels may be declining during the time of maternal recognition of pregnancy. It may be prudent to collect daily samples for at least 2 days or wait until after day 16 to collect a single sample after the time of MRP.

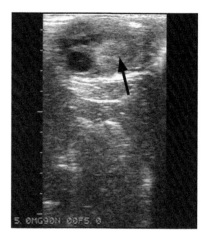

Figure 14-8. Small corpus luteum in a pregnant recipient mare (arrow).

Endometrial Cysts

Young recipient mares should not have endometrial cysts. However, if one or more cysts are present, the location and size should be recorded during ultrasound examinations performed prior to the mare receiving an embryo. Consequently, a cyst will not be confused with an embryonic vesicle during an early pregnancy examination (Figure 14-9).

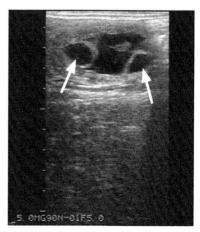

Figure 14-9. Endometrial cysts in a pregnant mare (arrows).

Uterine Fluid

The presence of free fluid within the uterine lumen is generally associated with inflammation and is usually incompatible with pregnancy. However, occasionally a small amount of free fluid is detected in the uterus of a pregnant mare and is often adjacent to the embryonic vesicle (Figure 14-10), or the embryo may be within the uterine fluid (Figure 14-11). Administration of systemic antibiotics should be considered in the event that bacterial endometritis is present and supplementation with progesterone or a progestin should also be considered. If the volume of fluid is significant or if the fluid is echogenic, the pregnancy will usually not survive.

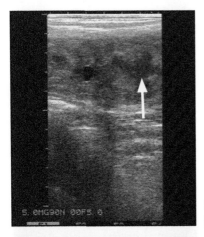

Figure 14-10. Free fluid within the uterus of a pregnant mare (arrow).

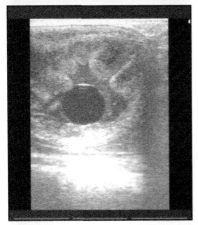

Figure 14-11. Embryo within a pool of uterine fluid.

Twins

Twins are a very uncommon and unexpected finding on ultrasound examination after transfer of a single embryo into a recipient mare. Several documented cases of twin embryos in embryo transfer recipient mares have been reported. In some cases two distinct embryonic vesicles have been detected (Figure 14-12), whereas in other cases two embryos, each with a heartbeat may be detected within one embryonic vesicle (Figure 14-13). In the former situation, standard procedures can be used to reduce one embryo and retain the other embryo. In the latter situation, the presence of twins is usually not detected until the recipient mare is examined for a heartbeat at day 25 to 35. Initial pregnancy examinations at day 11 to 16 would have revealed a single embryonic vesicle. It is usually not possible to eliminate one embryo and save the second embryo when twins occupy the same vesicle.

Unfortunately, not all embryo transfer pregnancies result in birth of a live foal. Early embryo loss may be identified during ultrasound examinations performed between days 11 and 50 of gestation. Loss may be recognized as an absence of a previously detected embryo or fetus, the presence of a small, underdeveloped embryo, absence of a heart beat in an embryo that is more than 25 days of age, loss of normal embryonic or fetal architecture, and/or detection of a degenerated embryo or fetus (Figure 14-14). It is recommended that the diagnosis of pregnancy loss be re-confirmed by a subsequent examination performed 24 to 48 hours after the initial examination, before a final diagnosis is made and prostaglandins administered.

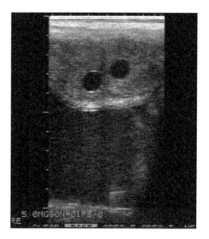

Figure 14-12. Ultrasonographic image of twin pregnancies, with individual embryonic vesicles separated slightly apart.

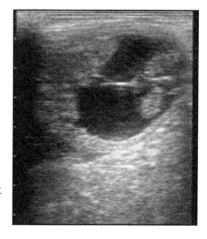

Figure 14-13. Ultrasonographic image of a 25 day pregnancy examination showing two embryos, each of which had a distinct heartbeat within one embryonic vesicle, in a recipient mare following transfer of a single embryo.

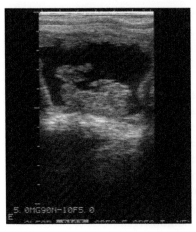

Figure 14-14. Pregnancy loss in a recipient mare. Note loss of normal embryonic structures.

Empty Trophoblastic Vesicle

An empty trophoblastic vesicle **(ETV)** is defined as an embryonic (trophoblastic) vesicle without an embryo proper. An embryo destined to form an ETV often exhibits normal early growth (i.e. day 11 to 16). Ultrasonographically, an ETV is recognized as a static oval or irregular embryonic structure without an embryo proper after day 25 of gestation (Figure 14-15). Empty trophoblastic vesicles do not form endometrial cups, even if the vesicle is still present in the uterus after day 35. Once an ETV has been confirmed, the recipient mare should be administered prostaglandins to cause luteolysis and allow for a return to estrus. It may be benficial to lavage the uterus of the mare after prostaglandin administration to remove embryonic membranes. Retention of embryonic membranes is often associated with accumulation of fluids in the uterus. This may be a result of immunologic recognition of foreign material (non-viable embryo tissue) in the uterine lumen by the mare.

In a retrospective study of 820 embryo transfers, a total of 20 empty trophoblastic vesicles were detected at day 25 following transfer. This represented 2.4% of all transfers and 3.3% of day 16 pregnancies.

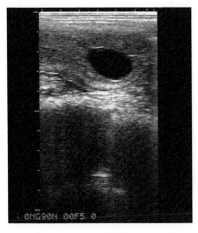

Figure 14-15. Ultrasonographic image of an empty trophoblastic vesicle (28 days after ovulation).

Recommended Reading

McCue PM, McKinnon AO. Pregnancy examination. In: Equine Reproduction. Second Edition. McKinnon AO, Squires EL, Vaala WE, Varner DD. (Eds). Wiley-Blackwell, Ames, Iowa. 2011, pp 1716-1727.

McCue, PM, Thayer J, Squires EL, Brinsko SP and Vanderwall DK. Twin pregnancies following transfer of single embryos in three mares: a case report. J. Equine Vet Sci 1998;18,832-834.

Vanderwall, DK, Squires, EL, Brinsko, SP, and McCue, PM. Diagnosis and management of abnormal embryonic development characterized by formation of an embryonic vesicle without an embryo in mares. Journal of the American Veterinary Medical Association, 2000;217(1):58-63.

Vullers A, Vullers F, Govaere G, Van Poucke M, Van Zeveren A, de Kruif A. Monozygotic twins after transfer of a single embryo. Reprod Dom Anim 2009;44, 131.

CHAPTER 15

PREGNANCY RATES
AFTER TRANSRER

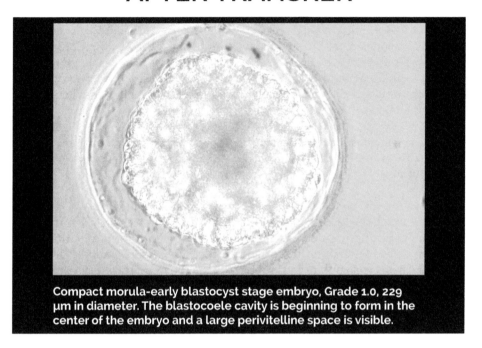

Compact morula-early blastocyst stage embryo, Grade 1.0, 229 µm in diameter. The blastocoele cavity is beginning to form in the center of the embryo and a large perivitelline space is visible.

Introduction

Pregnancy rate after transfer, pregnancy loss rate, and live foal rate are key statistics used to evaluate the success of an embryo transfer program. Pregnancy data are difficult to compare between different publications, embryo transfer centers and years because of differences in how results are reported, as some programs report any pregnancy achieved in a recipient mare while other programs report day 16 or 25 or 35 pregnancy rates or only live foal rate.

Pregnancy Rate after Transfer

A total of 1,063 client owned embryos were transferred at the Equine Reproduction Laboratory, Colorado State University between 2004 and 2013. An overall pregnancy rate at day 16 of 74.9% was achieved during that time period, which included data from all years, all embryos, of all grades, both fresh and cooled-transported embryos, and transfer results of all clinicians combined. In 2013, an overall pregnancy rate of 82.3% was attained.

Several strategic adjustments were made in the CSU embryo transfer program between 2010 and 2013 which have contributed to an overall improvement in pregnancy rates.

• Uterine culture and endometrial cytology examinations were performed on all recipient mares during their first heat cycle after arrival. Approximately 5 to 10 percent of recipient mares are identified each year with subclinical endometritis as defined by either bacterial growth on culture and/or the presence of white blood cells (neutrophils) on cytology. Affected mares are treated and re-cultured the next heat cycle. If they still have either a positive culture or a positive cytology, they were not used as a recipient.
• Mares receiving embryos were immediately placed back into their original herd instead of being moved into a "pregnant mare" herd with new mare additions and removals occurring daily. The goal was to reduce social stress on the recipient mares.
• The transfer procedure itself was modified with a goal of minimum manipulations of the uterus per rectum after the Cassou gun or pipette was passed throught the cervix.

Pregnancy Rate – Embryo Grade

Pregnancy rates for Grade 1 and 2 embryos are generally not different and are both higher than the pregnancy rate for Grades 3 and 4 embryos (Table 15-1).

Table 15 - 1.
Pregnancy rate at day 16 compared by grade and year.

Embryo Grade	2011 Season		2005-2010	
	(n)	Pregnancy Rate	(n)	Pregnancy Rate
1	78	80.7%	806	77.0%
2	5	100.0%	105	66.6%
3	2	50.0%	67	55.2%

Pregnancy rates were not different following transfer of fresh Grade 1 embryos than following transfer of Grade 1 embryos that had been cooled and transported for 12 to 24 hours in a passive cooling system (Table 15-2). A decrease in pregnancy rate was noted following transfer of lesser quality embryos that had been cooled and transported.

Table 15-2.
Day 16 pregnancy rates for equine embryos by Grade and status (fresh vs. cooled).

Embryo Grade	Fresh Embryos		Cooled Embryos	
	(n)	Pregnancy Rate	(n)	Pregnancy Rate
1	639	76.3%	232	76.2%
2	53	79.2%	48	60.4%
3 & 4	80	56.2%	30	53.3%

There was a significant difference ($p < 0.05$) in the day 16 pregnancy rate following transfer of embryos of different sizes (Table 15-3).The lowest pregnancy rates were from embryos < 200 μm and embryos 1,000 to 1,500 μm in diameter. It was postulated that the lower pregnancy rate for small embryos was not associated with embryo diameter *per se*, but more likely due to issues of abnormal embryonic development that ultimately resulted in the presence of a small embryo at the time of collection. The lower pregnancy rate for embryos 1,000 to 1,500 μm in diameter may have been due to damage to the embryo during collection, handling, washing or transfer.

Table 15-3.
Day 16 pregnancy rates for equine embryos of various sizes after transfer into recipient mares.

Embryo Size (μm)	(N)	Pregnancy Rate (%)
< 200	174	63.0[a]
200 to 399	388	77.3[b]
400 to 599	234	75.0[b]
600 to 799	130	78.0[b]
800 to 999	82	80.4[b]
1,000 to 1,500	48	69.0[a]
> 1,500	10	70.0[a,b]

Difference in superscript within a column indicates a significant difference in pregnancy rates ($p < 0.05$)

Pregnancy Rate – Transfer Clinician
A difference in pregnancy rates between clinicians within an embryo transfer center has been noted previously. Pregnancy rates at day 16 ranged from 70% to 91.8% for individual clinicians within the ET program at Colorado State University in 2013.

Pregnancy Rate – Other Embryo Transfer Centers

Pregnancy rates for other large embryo transfer programs are presented in Table 15-4.

Table 15-4.
Pregnancy rates after nonsurgical embryo transfer from several commercial embryo transfer programs throughout the world.

# Transfers	Pregnancy Rate (%)	Location	Reference
123	82.9%	USA	Foss et al., 1999
277	71.1%	Argentina	Riera, 2011
136	80.0%	Northern Ireland	Meadows et al, 2000
511	74.8%	Brazil	Fleury and Alvarenga, 1999
313	65.8%	Germany	Sánchez et al., 2005
212	79.6%	Italy	Panzani et al., 2009

Pregnancy Loss

Unfortunately, not all pregnant recipient mares remain pregnant and deliver a live foal. The highest rate of pregnancy loss is prior to day 50 in mares. A retrospective study of embryo transfer pregnancies at CSU revealed that 2.2% of pregnancies were lost between day of first detection (usually day 11) and day 16. Subsequently, 5.7% of the remaining pregnancies were lost between day 16 and 25, while an additional 2.5% were lost between day 25 and 35. The loss rate between day 35 and 50 was 0.8%. The total embryonic loss rate from day 11 to day 50 was 11.2%. A previous study reported a pregnancy loss rate of 15.5% between day 12 and day 50 for embryo transfer recipient mares.

Live Foal Rates

Limited data are available evaluating pregnancy outcome (i.e. live foal rates) in embryo transfer recipient mares. A retrospective study evaluated pregnancy outcome in mares carrying their own pregnancy with live foal rates following embryo transfer. A live healthy foal was born from 116 of 134 (86.6%) mares pregnant at day 16 carrying their own foal and 144 of 171 (84.2%) embryo transfer recipients pregnant at day 16 (p>0.05). No significant difference was noted in pregnancy outcome for recipient mares carrying pregnancies from young versus old embryo donor mares once a pregnancy had been diagnosed at day 16 pose-ovulation. The live foal rate for young recipient mares carrying pregnancies from older (> 15 years of age) donor mares (85.4%) was not significantly different (p>0.05) than that of older mares carrying their own pregnancy (79.4%).

Ultimately, the live foal rate was not significantly different between embryo transfer recipients and mares carrying their own foal once pregnancy was confirmed at day 16. In addition, the rate of pregnancy loss from day 16 to term was not significantly affected by age of the biological dam.

Summary

Multiple factors attribute to the success of an equine embryo transfer program. Attention to detail, consistency and dedication are required to achieve outstanding transfer success rates. Table 15-5 presents what we believe are high but achievable day 16 pregnancy rates following nonsurgical transfer in a commercial program.

Table 15-5.
Achievable pregnancy rates for nonsurgical embryo transfers performed in a commercial program.

Pregnancy Rate	Evaluation	Comments
≥ 90%	Outstanding	Difficult to consistently achieve with large numbers of transfers
80-90%	Excellent	Achievable with effort
75-80%	Very Good	A solid goal
70-75%	Good	Work on details
60-70%	Fair	Need to improve
< 60%	Marginal	Need significant improvement

Recommended Reading

Carnevale EM, Ramirez RJ, Squires EL, Alvarenga MA, Vanderwall DK, McCue PM. Factors affecting pregnancy rates and early embryonic death after equine embryo transfer. Theriogenology 2000;54:965-979.

Fleury JJ, Alvarenga MA. Effects of collection day on embryo recovery and pregnancy rates in a nonsurgical equine embryo transfer program. Theriogenology 1999; 51:261.

Foss R, Wirth N, Schiltz P, Jones J. Nonsurgical embryo transfer in a private practice (1998), in Proceedings. Am Assoc Equine Pract 1999; 45:210-212.

Hartman D. Embryo Transfer. In: Equine Reproduction. Second Edition. McKinnon AO, Squires EL, Vaala WE, Varner DD (Eds). Wiley-Blackwell, Ames, Iowa. 2011, pp 2871-2879.

Jasko DJ. Comparison of pregnancy rates following transfer of Day 8 equine embryos using various transfer devices. Theriogenology 2002; 58:713-716.

Meadows S, Lisa H, Welsh C. Factors affecting embryo recovery, embryo development and pregnancy rate in a commercial embryo transfer programme. Havemeyer Foundation Monograph Series 2000; 1:61-62.

Panzani D, Crisci A, Rota A, Camillo F. Effect of day of transfer and treatment administration on the recipient on pregnancy rates after equine embryo transfer. Vet Res Commun 2009; 33:S113-S116.

Riera FL. Equine embryo transfer. In: Samper JC, (ed). Equine breeding management and artificial insemination, Second edition. St Louis: Saunders Elsevier 2009; 185-199.

Riera F. General techniques and organization of large commercial embryo transfer programs. Clinical Theriogenology 2011; 3:318-324.

Sánchez R, Gomes I, Ramos H, Alvarenga MA, Carmo TM. Use of deep uterine low dose insemination of frozen and cooled stallion semen in a commercial embryo transfer programme. Havemeyer Foundation Monograph 2005; 14:103-104.

CHAPTER 16

FACTORS AFFECTING PREGNANCY RATES

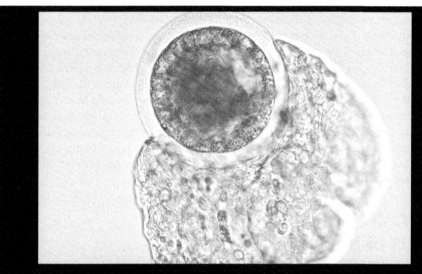

Early blastocyst stage embryo, Grade 1.0, 160 μm in diameter. A mass of cumulus cells is adherent to the zona pellucida. (courtesy of Dr. Hunter Ortis)

Introduction

In order to maximize the success of an equine embryo transfer program it is essential to know the factors that affect pregnancy rates. Factors affecting transfer success include embryo quality, age and reproductive status of the donor mare, technician and method of transfer, recipient quality, synchrony of the recipient and donor, season, and other factors.

Embryo Factors

Embryo age, size, developmental stage and quality can all affect pregnancy rates after transfer. A majority of equine embryos are collected seven or eight days after ovulation. Previous studies have reported that pregnancy rates for six, seven or eight-day-old embryos are similar as long as the size and developmental stage of the embryo matches the age of the embryo. For example, an embryo collected 8 days after ovulation should be an expanded blastocyst that is > 500 μm in diameter. A morula-stage embryo < 200 μm in diameter collected on day 8 would be considered delayed in development and transfer of the embryo may be associated with a reduced pregnancy rate or increased embryo loss rate. The quality of an embryo can also affect pregnancy rate after transfer. A majority of embryos collected from mares are Grade 1 (excellent quality) or Grade 2 (good quality). Embryos of lesser quality are associated with a decreased pregnancy rate or increased embryo loss rate.

Age and Reproductive Status of the Donor Mare

The age and reproductive health of the donor not only affect the ability to obtain an embryo, but can also impact pregnancy rates after transfer. It is essential that an owner understand the potential for reduced efficiency of an older donor mare in an embryo transfer program. The owner can then decide whether or not to keep an older mare in an embryo transfer program, allow the mare to attempt to carry her own foal to term or switch the mare to an assisted reproduction program. Many older mares that repeatedly fail to provide an embryo can become efficient donors of oocytes. Oocytes recovered from old mares can be transferred into the oviduct of a recipient that has been inseminated (oocyte transfer) or the oocyte can be injected with a spermatozoon (intra-cytoplasmic sperm injection) and the resulting embryo transferred into a recipient.

Common age related factors that result in decreased reproductive efficiency in mares include ovulation failure, mating-induced endometritis, infectious endometritis, endometrosis, and uterine cyst formation.

Two-year-old mares are occasionally used as embryo donors. Generally these are performance mares that are taken out of training long enough to be bred and have an embryo collected or young mares that have sustained a physical injury. Embryo recovery rates are low early in the two-year-old year of a donor, but increase later that season. Pregnancy rates after transfer are acceptable if an embryo can be obtained from a two-year-old. Stress of competition and training may impact embryo recovery.

Technician and Method of Transfer

The person performing a nonsurgical embryo transfer may have a dramatic influence on transfer success. Problem areas include: 1) handling the embryo, 2) loading the embryo into the Cassou gun, 3) passage of the Cassou gun or pipette through the cervix, 4) trauma during manipulation of the gun within the uterus. Training, practice and a dedication to success are keys to the success of individual transfer technicians.

Recipient Factors

The recipient mare is one of the most important factors affecting pregnancy rates after nonsurgical embryo transfer. Recipients can be provided by the owner of the donor mare or provided by the embryo transfer center. Strict quality control must be enforced when selecting a recipient for transfer, no matter what the source. An ideal recipient would be young (3 to 12 years of age), in good physical condition, easy to handle, and possess a gentle disposition. Maiden or open mares that have had foals previously make good recipient candidates. Older mares, mares in poor health, fractious mares, and barren mares are poor candidates as embryo recipients.

Pregnancy rates are higher if an embryo is transferred into a cycling recipient mare than into a hormone-treated acyclic mare. Consequently, recipient mares are placed under a stimulatory artificial photoperiod in early December (Northern Hemisphere) to stimulate follicular development and advance the first ovulation of the year. Occasionally a lack of cycling recipients necessitates the use of hormone-treated anestrous or ovariectomized mares as recipients. Transitional mares that have had some exposure to estradiol (i.e. follicles ≥ 25 mm and/or endometrial edema) make better recipients than mares in deep seasonal anestrus. Mares that have had their ovaries removed relatively recently (i.e. within 6 months) make better recipients than long-term ovariectomized mares.

Administration of 5 to 10 mg of estradiol-17β for 2 to 3 days followed by treatment with progesterone (200 mg, intramuscularly once daily) or altrenogest (0.044 mg/kg, orally once daily) can successfully prepare a non-cycling mare to receive an embryo. Exogenous hormone therapy should be timed to initiate progesterone therapy 1 to 2 days after ovulation of the donor mare. Progesterone therapy would need to continue until either accessory corpora lutea form or until after the placenta takes over progesterone production.

Recipient mares that do not become pregnant after the first transfer may receive a second embryo or occasionally a third embryo during a given breeding season. Clinical data has shown that the pregnancy rates for mares receiving their first or second embryo of a breeding season are not significantly different. However, pregnancy rate may be decreased if a original recipient mare receives a third embryo in a single season. Consequently, it is recommended that a mare only receive a maximum of 2 embryos per year, if possible. Recipient mares that accumulate a large volume of fluid in their uterus after receiving an embryo and mares that lose a pregnancy after day 35 (i.e. after endometrial cup formation) are not used as a recipient again that season.

Stress can have an adverse effect on pregnancy rates in recipient mares. Minimizing stress by maintaining a good herd health program, adequate nutrition, providing shelter and free access to fresh water should be standard in an embryo transfer program. Pregnancy rates are better for recipients that are gaining weight than for mares losing weight.

Another important consideration is to keep a recipient mare with her herd mates after transfer. Social stress associated with moving a mare into a new herd may adversely affect pregnancy rates.

Synchrony of the Recipient
A recipient mare must ovulate close to the day of the donor mare in order to achieve maximum pregnancy rates. Studies have shown that good pregnancy rates are possible if the recipient ovulates in a window from one day before the donor (+1) to 3 days after the donor (-3). Since most donor mares are flushed 7 or 8 days after ovulation, another way of achieving adequate donor-recipient synchrony is to select a recipient that ovulated 4 to 8 days prior to the collection day.

The non-steroidal anti-inflammatory drug meclofenamic acid has been evaluated as a means of utilizing recipient mares that are outside of the traditional window of acceptable synchrony with the donor mare. Administration of 1 g of meclofenamic acid orally once per day resulted in pregnancies being achieved when embryos were transferred into recipients that had ovulated 3, 4 or 5 days prior to the donor mare.

Season
It is not clear if a true seasonal effect exists on pregnancy rate after transfer. The issue is confounded by effects of environmental temperature and exposure on fertility of the donor mare, availability of good quality recipients throughout the breeding season, acquisition of new recipients during the middle of the season, and other factors. Anecdotal evidence suggests that pregnancy rates after transfer may be lower during excessively hot periods.

Recommended Reading

Carnevale EM, Ramirez RJ, Squires EL, Alvarenga MA, Vanderwall DK, McCue PM. Factors affecting pregnancy rates and early embryonic death after equine embryo transfer. Theriogenology 2000; 54:965-979.

Riera F. Systematic approach to efficiency problems in an embryo transfer program. Clinical Theriogenology 2011; 3:325-341.

Squires EL, Imel KJ, Iuliano MF, Shideler RK. Factors affecting reproductive efficiency in an equine embryo transfer programme. J Reprod Fert 1982; Suppl 32:409-414.

CHAPTER 17

DISEASE TRANSMISSION

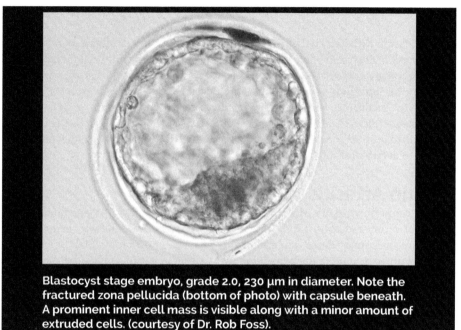

Blastocyst stage embryo, grade 2.0, 230 μm in diameter. Note the fractured zona pellucida (bottom of photo) with capsule beneath. A prominent inner cell mass is visible along with a minor amount of extruded cells. (courtesy of Dr. Rob Foss).

Introduction

Prevention of transmission of pathogenic organisms to the recipient mare is critical to the success of an embryo transfer program. Incorporation of sterile equipment, aseptic techniques, sanitary handling and detail-oriented reproductive management are imperative.

Limited data exists for transmission of pathogenic organisms to a recipient mare following transfer of an in vivo produced equine embryo. Disease pathogens that could potentially be transmitted to a recipient mare via an infected embryo include bacterial, fungal and viral organisms.

Contamination with bacterial or fungal organisms may potentially be recognized clinically by: 1) detection of an abnormal uterine environment prior to breeding by culture, cytology or biopsy, 2) presence of echogenic fluid in the uterus after breeding (rule out non-infectious persistent mating-induced endometritis), 3) presence of debris in the media recovered during the embryo collection procedure, or 4) presence of debris adhered to the embryo. Contamination with a viral agent, such as equine arteritis virus (EAV) or equine herpesvirus type-1 **(EHV-1)**, would be much more difficult to detect clinically.

Equine Arteritis Virus (EAV)

A study was performed in which donor mares vaccinated against EAV and donor mares not vaccinated against EAV were inseminated with EAV-infective semen. Embryo recovery procedures were performed 7 days after ovulation. Embryos were washed 5 times in embryo flush medium, two times in trypsin, and 5 more times in embryo flush medium prior to transfer. Embryo flush media and wash fluid were evaluated for EAV by virus isolation and real-time PCR. Recipient mares were monitored for development of virus neutralizing antibody titers (seroconversion). Results of the study indicated that uterine flush fluid from 9 of 15 non-vaccinated and 2 of 11 vaccinated donor mares were positive for presence of equine arteritis virus. The washing protocol did not eliminate EAV from all embryos and two recipients seroconverted after receiving an embryo. The study concluded that there may be a risk of transmission of EAV following transfer of an embryo recovered from a mare inseminated with EAV infective semen.

Equine Herpes Virus 1 (EHV-1)

Another study evaluated the potential risk of transmission of equine herpesvirus 1 by embryo transfer. Embryos collected from donor mares were exposed to EHV-1 *in vitro* for 24 hours before being washed 10 times in sterile phosphate-buffered saline (PBS) containing 0.4% BSA, antibiotics and an antimycotic agent in accordance with recommendations of the International Embryo Transfer Society (IETS). Trypsin washes were not used in this study. The PBS wash solutions and embryos were subsequently evaluated for presence of EHV-1. Virus was detected in the first 5 wash solutions, but was absent in the last 5 wash solutions. Virus was detected in 7 of 10 embryos after washing was completed, suggesting that EHV-1 could either attach to the zona pellucida or capsule, or had penetrated the embryo.

Apparently the only report of natural contamination of an embryo with EHV-1 has been the detection of virus in a single embryo collected from a clinically healthy donor mare.

Risk Potential for Disease Transmission

In contrast to the horse, considerable research has been performed in cattle and other livestock species to assess the potential for disease transmission via *in vivo* and *in vitro* produced embryos. In general, the risk of transmission of a viral agent from *in vivo* derived embryos has been considered to be very low.

The risk for disease transmission via equine embryos depends on a combination of exposure potential, breeding management practices, embryo handling procedures, transfer technique and management of the recipient mare. Management practices that would reduce the risk of disease transmission include vaccination of donor mares, monitoring health status of the donor mare, knowledge of the EAV status of the stallion, evaluation of the donor mare after breeding, evaluation of the embryo collection medium and the embryo, and thorough washing of the embryo.

Embryo Processing (Bovine)

Embryo processing for bovine embryos recommended by the IETS is as follows:
• Evaluate the embryo under a stereomicroscope using at least 50x magnification to observe defects and presence of debris adhering to the zona pellucida.
• Remove debris adherent to the zona pellucida by repeated pipetting.
• Wash embryos by passage through at least 10 aliquots of sterile, buffered saline medium containing 0.4% bovine serum albumin (BSA) and broad spectrum antibiotics.
• Two trypsin treatments may be incorporated into the wash protocol. The embryo should be washed 5 times in BSA, and then passed through 2 aliquots of sterile 0.25% trypsin in a buffered saline solution without Ca^{2+} or Mg^{2+}, but with antibiotics, for a total exposure of 60 to 90 seconds. After the trypsin treatments, the embryo is passed through the remaining 5 BSA washes with 2% serum or 0.4% BSA to serve as a substrate to remove the remaining enzymatic activity of the trypsin. Note: exposure of equine embryos to 0.2% trypsin has been reported to result in a "sticky" capsule that may complicate embryo handling.
• Each wash must involve at least a 100-fold dilution of the previous wash.
• Fresh, sterile pipettes should be used to transfer embryos between each well.
• Embryos should be gently stirred within each well.
• Embryos should be re-examined after washing to ensure that the zona is still intact and free of adherent material.

Additional Considerations for Equine Embryos

If a significant amount of debris is present in the embryo recovery media or if debris is adhered to the embryo, it may be prudent to administer antibiotics to the recipient mare due to the potential for bacterial contamination. Clinical experience has shown that the risk of development of bacterial endometritis in the recipient mare is high after transfer of an embryo covered with debris.

If potential exists for transmission of EAV from an embryo collected from an infected donor mare, the recipient mare should be isolated from the rest of the herd to prevent horizontal transmission of the virus. It may be beneficial to vaccinate all recipient mares against EAV to minimize the potential for viral transmission.

Embryos cryopreserved in unsealed vials or straws have the theoretical potential to be contaminated with pathogenic microorganisms if the liquid nitrogen is contaminated. Proper sealing of straws or other containers will reduce or eliminate the potential for contamination.

Summary

There is a potential for transfer of bacterial, fungal or viral organisms during embryo transfer. The risk can be minimized by proper reproductive management of the donor and recipient mares and washing the embryo. There is no universal disinfection protocol that can render all embryos free from all potentially pathogenic microorganisms.

Recommended Reading

Bielanski A. Disinfection procedures for controlling microorganisms in the semen and embryos of humans and farm animals. Theriogenology 2007; 68:1-22.

Broaddus CC, Balasuriya UBR, Timoney PJ, White JLR, Makloski C, Torrisi K, Payton M, Holyoak GR. Infection of embryos following insemination of donor mares with equine arteritis virus infective semen. Theriogenology 2011; 76:47-60.

Hebia I, Fiéni F, Duchamp G, Destrumelle S, Pellerin J-L, Zientara S, Vautherot J-F, Bruyas J-F. Potential risk of equine herpes virus 1 (EHV-1) transmission by equine embryo transfer. Theriogenology 2007; 67:1485-1491.

Stringfellow DA. Recommendations for the sanitary handling of in-vivo-derived embryos. In: Stringfellow DA and Seidel SM (eds), Manual of the International Embryo Transfer Society. Third edition. IETS, Savoy, Illinois; 1998, pp. 79-84.

Wrathall AE, Simmons HA, Van Soom A. Evaluation of risks of viral transmission to recipients of bovine embryos arising from fertilization with virus-infected semen. Theriogenology 2006; 65:247-274.

CHAPTER 18

INTERNATIONAL TRANSPORT OF EMBRYOS

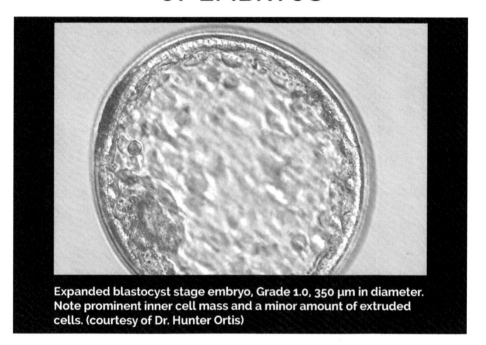

Expanded blastocyst stage embryo, Grade 1.0, 350 μm in diameter. Note prominent inner cell mass and a minor amount of extruded cells. (courtesy of Dr. Hunter Ortis)

Introduction

Equine embryos are transported internationally to take advantage of economic markets in another country and to reduce the cost and safety risk associated with transport of live horses. In some geographic regions, such as within the European Union, an embryo collected on a breeding farm or clinic in one country may be transported to a specialty reproduction center in another country for transfer into a recipient mare.

Transport Options

Equine embryos may be cooled and transported internationally by a private courier service (same day delivery) or by a commercial carrier (next-day delivery) if the final destination is within a reasonable distance and regulations for export/import are not prohibitive.

Shipment of embryos from one country to another can be a significant challenge. Embryos may be held up in customs for days, which would preclude transport of fresh-cooled embryos, and require transport of cryopreserved embryos in a liquid nitrogen (LN2) container, such as a vapor (dry) shipping container (Figure 18-1). A vapor shipping container is "charged" by filling the container with LN2, allowing time for LN2 to be absorbed into the wall of the container and then removing the excess liquid prior to use. Consequently, a vapor container is not considered as hazardous and may be placed on commercial flights for transport. The vapor shipping container can maintain temperature close to -196° C for 7 or more days.

An experienced broker, agent or courier service may be valuable to streamline international transport of embryos. The broker can verify that all documents are

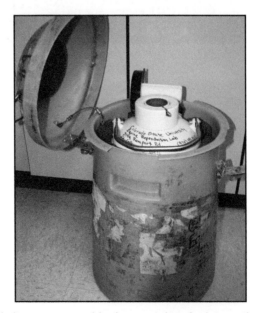

Figure 18-1. Liquid nitrogen vapor shipping container for international transport of embryos. The aluminum tank is housed within an outer plastic case.

complete and secure a direct flight to the correct airport in the importing country. On the receiving end, a broker can make sure the embryo container clears customs and is delivered safely to the consignee.

Regulations

International transport of embryos and other biologic material is often regulated to limit the potential for transmission of pathogenic disease agents. The disease risk associated with importation of embryos has been determined to be negligible in cattle, provided that embryos are handled in accordance with guidelines published by the International Embryo Transfer Society **(IETS)**. Equine breeding managers, veterinarians, technicians and others involved in the reproductive management of the donor mare, embryo collection, processing, cryopreservation, transport, and transfer into the recipient mare should all be responsible for due diligence in hygiene and disease prevention.

It is imperative that specific regulations regarding international transport of embryos be understood well in advance of embryo collection. Regulations should be followed precisely and accurate records maintained in order to ship an embryo to another country. An import permit should be acquired by the person importing the embryo (consignee). The permit will outline specific requirements for importation of equine embryos into that country. Many countries do not have specific regulations for export or import of equine embryos. Consequently, it is important to be aware of the individual requirements of an importing country since regulations may vary considerably among counties.

An International Animal Health Certificate signed by an accredited veterinarian and/ or inspector of the central veterinary service of the country of origin may be required to accompany the embryo shipment. Additional import or export requirements are often specific for a country or economic/political union (i.e. the European Union). General requirements may include some or all of the following (or more):
1. International Animal Health Certificate for the embryo
   a. Clear description of shipment
   b. Import permit number
   c. Name of exporting country
   d. Health Certificate issue and expiration dates
   e. Name and address and contact information of exporter or consignor of the embryo
   f. Registered name and registration number of the donor mare
   g. Registered name and registration number of the semen donor or stallion
   h. Breed of mares and stallion
   i. Number of straws/embryos
   j. Date of collection
   k. Identification of straw
   l. Name, address and contact information of embryo collection or processing center or team
   m. Registration number of embryo collection or processing center or team
   n. Number of containers
   o. Official seal number

p. Name, address and contact information of importer or consignee of the embryo

q. Name and address of destination of the embryo

r. Transportation means

s. Date and place of embarkation from the country of origin

t. Date and place of entry into the country of destination

2. Name, license number and address of veterinarian in charge of embryo collection.

3. Registration and inspection of the embryo collection and processing center may be required.

4. Isolation of donor mares from other horses for a specific period of time at an approved collection center prior to embryo collection may be required.

5. Certification that the collection center is free of specific disease pathogens or inspection of the donors and other horses on the premises for clinical signs of specific transmissible equine diseases may be required. Certification that no horses have shown signs of specific diseases for a designated time period prior to embryo collection may be required.

6. Diagnostic tests for specific disease pathogens may be required on the donor mare within a specific time interval prior to embryo collection. It may be required that samples be collected by an accredited or approved veterinarian and submitted to an official approved laboratory.

7. Vaccination of the donor mares against specific pathogenic organisms may be required.

8. Verification of health status or testing of stallions or semen used for breeding the donor mare may be required.

9. It may be required that the donor mare and stallion not be used for live or natural cover for a specific period of time prior to embryo collection.

10. It may be required that the site of embryo collection, processing and storage be separated from other parts of the premises.

11. It may be required that equipment used to collect, handle, wash, cryopreserve and store embryos be new, disposable or properly sterilized prior to use.

12. It may be required that all biological products of animal origin used for the collection, processing and storage of embryos be free of microorganisms. Additional requirements for fetal bovine serum or serum albumin may be present.

13. It may be required to confirm that care was taken to prevent contamination during the procedures used for the production and storage of embryos.

14. Specific procedures to handle and wash the embryo may be required, such as the guidelines of the International Embryo Transfer Society (IETS). It may be required that the zona pellucida be intact and that the embryo be free of adherent material.

15. It may be required that embryos are stored in new or cleaned and disinfected containers with first-use liquid nitrogen. A specific storage time prior to embarkation may be required, during which time the donor mares are evaluated for evidence of clinical transmissible diseases.

16. Specific forms may be required for embryo identification.

17. Embryos may be required to be in sealed sterile straws or pipettes, each clearly marked with identification of the donor mare, collection date and embryo collection center.

18. The shipment container is usually inspected and sealed by an official of the exporting country.

19. Shipment containers may be required to be disinfected at the airport in the exporting country prior to departure and again on arrival into the importing country under official supervision.

20. Accurate records will be required.

Information Resources

Information on international transport of embryos and regulatory forms are available on a variety of web sites, including:

Importation of Equine Embryos into Australia:
http://www.daff.gov.au/aqis/import/biological/products-foodstuffs

Import of Equine Embryos into the European Union:
http://ec.europa.eu/food/animal/semen_ova/equine/index_en.htm

Importation of Equine Embryos into the United States:
http://www.aphis.usda.gov/import_export/animals/equine_dog_semen.shtml

Recommended Reading

Bishop E. Import and export of embryos. In: Equine Reproduction, Second Edition. Edited by McKinnon AO, Squires EL, Vaala WE, Varner DD. Wiley-Blackwell Publishing Ltd, 2011, pp. 2,921-2,923.

OIE (World Organization for Animal Health). Import risk analysis. Terrestrial Animal Health Code. OIE (World Organization for Animal Health), Paris, 2010.

Stringfellow DA, Seidel SM. Manual of the International Embryo Transfer Society, Third Edition. International Embryo Transfer Society, Savoy, Illinois, 1998.

CHAPTER 19

RELATED EMBRYO TECHNOLOGIES

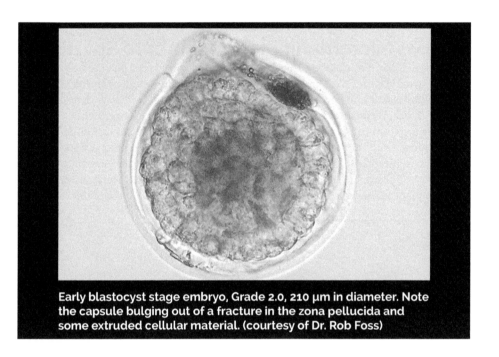

Early blastocyst stage embryo, Grade 2.0, 210 µm in diameter. Note the capsule bulging out of a fracture in the zona pellucida and some extruded cellular material. (courtesy of Dr. Rob Foss)

Introduction

Several advanced assisted reproduction procedures require transfer of embryos into recipient mares. In some instances the original embryo may be produced *in vivo* and in other cases the embryo may be produced *in vitro* by intra-cytoplasmic sperm injection **(ICSI)** or somatic cell nuclear transfer **(NT)**. Conventional *in vitro* fertilization **(IVF)** is still problematic in the horse, with only 2 live foals born in France reported in 1991. The IVF foals were produced from *in vivo* matured oocytes collected from gonadotropin-stimulated donor mares. There are currently no reports of live foals produced from *in vitro* matured oocytes and conventional IVF.

Embryo Micromanipulation (Embryo Splitting)

Transection of day 6 morula or early blastocyst stage embryos has been used to create identical twins (Figures 19-1 and 19-2). In the original equine studies, the bisected demi-embryos were transferred surgically into the uterus of separate synchronized recipient mares. Ultimately, the low success rate for production of live healthy twin foals by embryo splitting is a limiting factor for incorporation of this technique into clinical practice. Additional studies are needed to optimize this technique since it could be a means of increasing the number of foals produced from a donor mare on a single cycle without superovulation. Alternatively, one demi-embryo could be transferred into a recipient mare and the other cryopreserved for transfer at a later date.

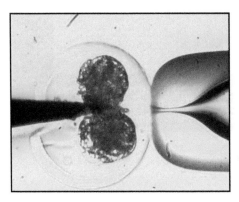

Figure 19-1. Transection of a bovine embryo held with suction from a micropipette using a fragment of a razor blade (from Williams et al., 1984).

Oocyte Transfer (OT)

Traditional oocyte transfer in the horse involves surgical transfer of a single oocyte into an inseminated recipient mare that has had her own oocyte removed. Fertilization, early embryonic development, and subsequent fetal development all occur within the recipient mare. In specific instances, transfer of multiple oocytes into the oviduct of an inseminated recipient mare may occur. The uterus of the recipient mare may be flushed 7 or 8 days after transfer and the recovered embryos evaluated and transferred individually into separate synchronized recipient mares that would hopefully carry the pregnancy to term.

The main application of OT followed by ET would be the emergency collection of multiple oocytes harvested from ovaries of a mare after euthanasia and the availability of a large number of motile spermatozoa from a fertile stallion for

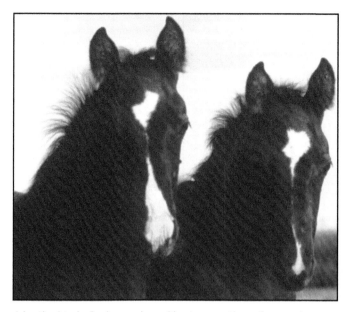

Figure 19-2. Identical twin foals produced by transection of an embryo.

traditional insemination of the OT recipient mare. Transfer of all oocytes into the oviduct of a single recipient would bypass the need for intra-cytoplasmic sperm injection **(ICSI)** of individual oocytes and *in vitro* culture. In contrast, ICSI would be more appropriate if a limited number of oocytes were collected and (especially) if the number of motile sperm was limited.

Oocyte collection and transfer is an option as a means of obtaining a pregnancy from an embryo donor that fails to provide an embryo after conventional uterine flush procedures.

Intra-Cytoplasmic Sperm Injection (ICSI)

Intra-cytoplasmic sperm injection (ICSI) is an advanced reproductive procedure in which a single spermatozoon is inserted into the cytoplasm of an oocyte that has been collected from an ovarian follicle and matured *in vitro* (Figure 19-3). The procedure has been used clinically to obtain pregnancies from 1) old mares with reproductive abnormalities that preclude normal *in vivo* fertilization or embryo development, 2) mares for which the number of motile spermatozoa available for insemination is very limited, and 3) oocytes harvested from mares following euthanasia.

Intra-cytoplasmic sperm injection allows for *in vitro* production of equine embryos and birth of live foals (Figure 19-4) bypassing the requirement for a spermatozoon to bind to and penetrate the zona pellucida of the equine oocyte, which has been a road block to the success of conventional IVF in the horse. ICSI also has the advantage over oocyte transfer in that ejaculates with a low number of motile spermatozoa or small portion of a straw of frozen semen can be used, the recipient's oocyte does not have to be removed, and there is no risk of post-mating endometritis in the recipient mare.

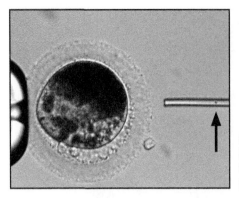

Figure 19-3. Intra-cytoplasmic sperm injection (ICSI) of an equine oocyte. Note the spermatozoon within the injection pipette (arrow).

It is now possible to ship oocytes to an ICSI facility and have the *in vitro* produced embryo sent back to the clinic that provided the original oocyte.

A motile spermatozoon can be used for ICSI from stallions with good or poor pregnancy rates in traditional breeding programs. In addition, fresh, cooled-transported, frozen-thawed spermatozoa, or even frozen epididymal sperm can be utilized successfully. Incorporation of the Piezo drill for ICSI, which produces a hole in the zona pelucida through which a sperm is subsequently injected, has significantly enhanced success rates.

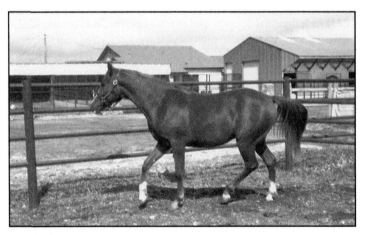

Figure 19-4. First horse born following intra-cytoplasmic sperm injection.

The injected oocyte may be transferred immediately into the oviduct of a recipient mare or may be cultured *in vitro* and embryo development observed. A cleavage-stage embryo (Figure 19-5) may be surgically transferred into the oviduct of a synchronized recipient mare or the embryo cultured for an additional 5 to 7 days (Figures 19-6 through 19-7) and transferred directly into the uterus of a recipient mare by a traditional non-surgical technique.

Embryonic development of *in vitro* produced equine embryos may be delayed in comparison to *in vivo* produced embryos. Consequently, a day 7 ICSI-derived embryo may have the optimal chance of success if transferred into a recipient mare that
152

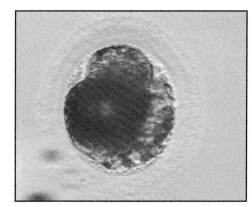

Figure 19-5. A cleavage-stage (2-cell) embryo 24 hours following ICSI.

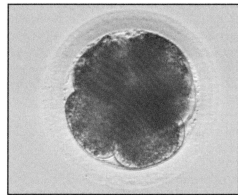

Figure 19-6. A four cell embryo developing *in vitro* two days after ICSI.

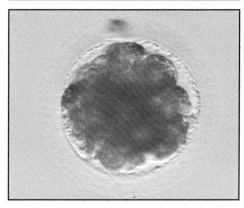

Figure 19-7. An 8-16 cell embryo developing *in vitro* four days after ICSI.

ovulated 5 days previously. In other words, the developmental stage of the embryo should be taken into account when selecting a recipient mare.

In vitro produced embryos produced outside of the traditional breeding season can also be cultured and subsequently cryopreserved at the late morula or early blastocyst stage. Embryos can be thawed (warmed) and transferred when a suitable synchronized recipient is available during the breeding season

Pregnancy rates after transfer of in vitro produced embryos ranged in one report from 25 to 72.7%. A live foal rate of 83% of established pregnancies was noted in that study.

Autogenous Transfer of ICSI Produced Embryos

Intracytoplasmic sperm injection may be used to produce embryos from oocytes collected from reproductively normal donor mares. In these instances, the limiting factor for successful reproduction has been sperm quality or quantity. Embryos generated by ICSI historically have been either transferred surgically into the oviduct of a recipient mare or non – surgically into the uterus of a recipient mare. A recent study has shown that ICSI – produced embryos can be cultured *in vitro* to a morula or early blastocyst stage and transferred non – surgically directly back into the uterus of the donor mare. The autogenous transfer technique has subsequently been used clinically to produce pregnancies in several privately owned mares.

Somatic Cell Nuclear Transfer (Cloning)

"Dolly", a lamb born in 1996, was the first mammal produced by nuclear transfer of an adult derived somatic cell. The first cloned equids, 3 mule foals and a horse foal, were born in 2003. The mule foals were produced by nuclear transfer from fetal somatic cells of a 45 day old fetus into *in vivo* matured oocytes. The recombined oocytes were activated and immediately surgically transferred into the oviducts of the surrogate mares.

In contrast, a cloned horse foal (Figure 19-8) was produced by nuclear transfer of adult somatic cells using *in vitro* matured oocytes as the recipient of the donor nuclei. Resulting embryos were cultured *in vitro* to the blastocyst stage before nonsurgical transfer into the uterus of the original donor mare.

Pregnancy and live foal rate following nonsurgical transfer of somatic cell nuclear transfer derived embryos is substantially less than that of ICSI or *in vivo* generated embryos. A recent report indicated that 11% of frozen-thawed cloned embryos result in pregnancies in recipient mares after transfer and that 23% of the pregnancies resulted in birth of a live foal.

Nuclear transfer has been touted as a means of preserving the genetics of valuable individual horses. Perhaps the most interesting clinical application of nuclear transfer is production of a stallion from somatic cells harvested from a gelding. The offspring should theoretically produce fertile spermatozoa as an adult stallion.

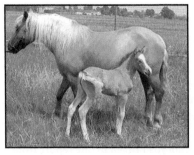

Figure 19-8. Photograph of a cloned foal born to its dam twin (courtesy of Dr. Cesare Galli).

Pre-Implantation Genetic Diagnoses (PGD)

Biopsy of an *in vivo* or *in vitro* produced equine embryo would allow preimplantation genetic diagnosis **(PGD)** for sex determination or detection of inherited genetic defects. Examples of inherited recessive genetic defects in horses that could potentially be identified in an equine embryo biopsy include hyperkalemic periodic paralysis **(HYPP)**, hereditary equine regional dermal asthenia **(HERDA)**, severe combined immunodeficiency disorder **(SCID)**, and cerebellar abiotrophy.

Theoretically, PGD could be performed on a single blastomere or a small number of trophoblast cells harvested from an embryo. Options for collection of an embryo biopsy include a microblade technique or aspiration of cells following penetration of the zona pellucid and capsule with a Piezo drill (Figure 19-9). Recent studies have shown that collection of cells by aspiration is associated with higher pregnancy rates after transfer than biopsy using a microblade.

The biopsied embryo can be 1) cultured *in vitro* prior to transfer if the PGD is performed immediately, 2) cryopreserved to allow time for PGD prior to a transfer decision, or 3) transferred immediately into a recipient. The latter option may entail a decision as to whether or not to allow the recipient to remain pregnant depending on results of the genetic testing.

Additional research is needed to optimize biopsy techniques, cryopreservation methods for biopsied embryos, and PGD of equine embryo biopsies.

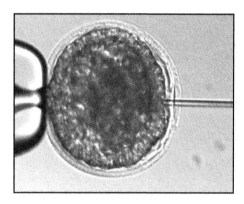

Figure 19-9. Collection of trophoblast cells from an early blastocyst stage embryo.

Recommended Reading

Allen WR, Pashen RL. Production of monozygotic (identical) horse twins by embryo micromanipulation. J Reprod Fertil 1984; 71:607-613.

Carnevale EM, Stokes JE, Rossini JB, Rodriguez JS. Autogenous transfers of intracytoplasmic sperm injection – produced equine embryos into oocyte donor uteri. Annual Convention American Association of Equine Practitioners 2013; 59; 200-203.

Galli C, Lagutina I, Crotti G, Colleoni S, Turini P, Ponderato N, Duchi R, Lazzari G. A cloned horse born to its dam twin. Nature 2003; 424:635.

Galli C, Colleoni S, Duchi R, Lagutina L, Lazzari G. Developmental competence of equine oocytes and embryos obtained by in vitro procedures ranging from in vitro maturation and ICSI to embryo culture, cryopreservation and somatic cell nuclear transfer. Animal Reprod Science 2007; 98:39-55.

Hinrichs K. Update on equine ICSI and cloning. Theriogenology 2005; 64:535-541.

Hinrichs K. Biopsy and vitrification of equine expanded blastocytes. Clinical Theriogenology 2011; 3:314-317.

Seidel GE, Cullingford, EL, Stokes JE, Carnevale, EM, McCue PM. Pregnancy rates following transfer of biopsied and/or vitrified equine embryos: evaluation of two biopsy techniques. Animal Reprod Sci 2010; 121S: 297-298.

Slade NP, Williams TJ, Squires EL, Seidel Jr. GE. Production of identical twin pregnancies by microsurgical bisection of equine embryos. Proc 10th Int Congr Anim Reprod AI II. 1984; 10:241.

Williams TJ, Elsden RP, Seidel Jr. GE. Pregnancy rates with bisected bovine embryos. Theriogenology 1984; 22:521-531.

Woods GL, White KL, Vanderwall DK, Li G-P, Aston KI, Bunch TD, Meerdo LN, Pate BJ. A mule cloned from fetal cells by nuclear transfer. Science 2003; 301:1063.

CHAPTER 20

FUTURE DIRECTIONS OF EQUINE EMBRYO TRANSFER

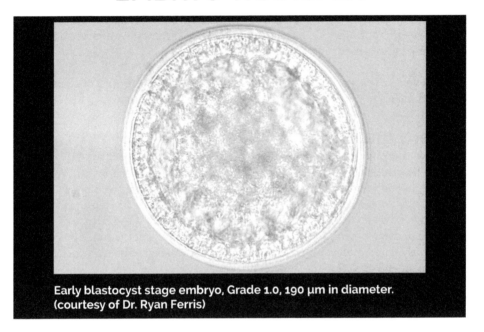

Early blastocyst stage embryo, Grade 1.0, 190 μm in diameter.
(courtesy of Dr. Ryan Ferris)

Introduction

Significant advancements have occurred in our scientific knowledge and clinical application of embryo transfer in horses over the past 40 years. Future research and technique development in embryo technologies will likely be aimed at four main areas: 1) enhancing embryo recovery rate by increasing ovulation rate (i.e. superovulation), 2) improved techniques for cooled storage and cryopreservation of embryos, 3) embryo biopsy for gender determination and genetic diagnosis, and 4) production of embryos through *in vitro* fertilization or intra-cytoplasmic sperm injection. Continued research in mare reproductive physiology and pathology will be critical to improving embryo recovery rates in problem mares. International markets for embryos are contingent on refining techniques for cryopreservation of embryos and optimizing pregnancy rates after transfer.

Outlined below are some areas of future research and potential growth of equine embryo transfer:

Superovulation

Mares typically only ovulate one follicle per estrous cycle spontaneously. As a consequence, the goal of an embryo recovery procedure is to collect one embryo per cycle, and only about 50 to 65% of cycles result in recovery of an embryo. Techniques to consistently increase the number of follicles that develop and ovulate synchronously would increase embryo recovery rate, improve the efficiency of embryo transfer per cycle, and potentially lower the cost of embryo transfer. There are currently no hormone products commercially available for enhancing follicular development and ovulation (i.e. superovulation).

Recombinant equine follicle stimulating hormone **(reFSH)** appears to have great potential in the horse. Unfortunately, reFSH is not yet approved for use in the horse. Other hormone therapies, such as pFSH, oFSH, eCG and GnRH have limited to no efficacy in enhancing ovulation rates in the mare. Research studies evaluating reFSH and eFSH have shown that embryo recovery can be increased 3 to 4 fold by inducing multiple ovulations in donor mares.

Early Pregnancy Factor

An immunosuppressive glycoprotein called "early pregnancy factor" **(EPF)**, first described in the mouse, has been reported in the mare. Early studies used the rosette inhibition test **(RIT)** to detect EPF, which was shown to increase in peripheral blood within 2 days after ovulation. Serum levels were reported to decrease in embryo donor mares within 2 days after flushing an embryo out of the uterus and increase in recipient mares within 2 to 3 days after receiving an embryo. It was noted that two patterns of EPF activity were evident in recipient mares that did not become pregnant after transfer. In some recipient mares, EPF activity remained low, suggesting that the embryo did not remain viable after transfer. In other mares, EPF activity increased 2 days after transfer, but subsequently decreased to non-pregnant levels by 5 days after transfer, suggesting that the embryos were initially viable after transfer and then died.

These studies suggest that early pregnancy factor is produced by the early developing embryo soon after fertilization while still in the oviduct and that EPF may be a useful marker for pregnancy and embryo viability. Development of an accurate and repeatable assay for EPF could be extremely valuable in the reproductive evaluation of a problem mare (i.e. did the mare ever become pregnant) and could potentially be used to determine if a viable embryo is present in the uterus prior to performing an embryo collection procedure.

Heat shock protein 10 (HSP-10), the putative early pregnancy factor, has been detected in equine embryos by immunohistochemistry. It remains to be determined if HSP-10 can be detected in the peripheral blood of pregnant mares.

Oviductal Abnormalities

Pathological issues with the equine oviduct are poorly understood and difficult to diagnose. As a consequence, subfertility due to oviductal blockage is usually underdiagnosed and therapies designed for treatment of oviductal blockage are often performed on mares without the benefit of a diagnostic test to confirm the actual presence of a blockage. Laparoscopic application of PGE_2 gel to the surface of the oviducts of infertile mares has been reported to result in a return to fertility in some mares. Clearly, additional controlled studies on both diagnostic techniques and therapeutic procedures are needed in this misunderstood area.

Cryopreservation of Embryos

Even though the first foal produced after transfer of a frozen-thawed embryo was born in 1982, cryopreservation of equine embryos for commercial use is still uncommon. The primary roadblock to clinical application is the decreased pregnancy rate following transfer of cryopreserved embryos compared to transfer success for fresh or cooled embryos. The fact that mares only donate one embryo per cycle leads to a high value and high expectation for each embryo. Successful superovulation would reduce the pressure associated with the collection and transfer of individual embryos. In addition, only small equine embryos (≤ 300 µm) have been successfully cryopreserved with reasonable success using current slow freezing or vitrification techniques. Superovulation and the ability to successfully cryopreserve larger equine embryos will lead to a dramatic expansion of the use of frozen embryos. This will, in turn, lead to more international marketing of equine genetics via frozen embryos.

Cryopreservation could also dramatically alter how recipient mares are utilized. An owner could wait until an embryo is actually recovered from an individual donor mare, then acquire a recipient for that particular embryo and have the embryo transferred at a time of year that is optimal.

Assisted Reproduction Technologies

Techniques to produce equine embryos in vitro, including intra-cytoplasmic sperm injection (**ICSI**) and somatic cell nuclear transfer (cloning) are now available on a limited basis to horse owners. Embryos produced *in vitro* and cultured to the morula or early blastocyst stage may be transferred non-surgically into the uterus of a recipient mare.

Other related techniques, such as oocyte collection on breeding farms or veterinary clinics and shipment of oocytes to a referral center for ICSI followed by shipment of embryos back to the original farm or clinic for non-surgical transfer into a recipient mare are now in full clinical use.

In vitro production and subsequent nonsurgical transfer of equine embryos are likely to become more common in the future. Sex selected semen may become incorporated into the fertilization process in the future, similar to what has happened in the cattle industry. However, efficiency of sperm sorting and enhancement of procedures for successful cryopreservation of sexed equine semen will need to be improved.

Future assisted reproduction programs will likely continue to rely on non-surgical transfer of in vitro derived embryos.

Pre-Implantation Genetic Diagnoses (PGD)

Understandably, the optimal goal of some horse breeders is to preselect the sex of an embryo by insemination of a donor mare with sex-sorted spermatozoa. Unfortunately, sex-sorting of equine semen is not currently commercially available. One alternative is to wait until day 65 to 70 of pregnancy and determine the sex of the fetus using transrectal ultrasonography. However, this is a long time to wait for information on whether or not to rebreed the donor mare or whether or not to maintain the pregnancy in the recipient mare.

Another alternative is to determine the sex of an early embryo by genetic testing of blastomeres or trophoblast cells collected by embryo biopsy. Clinical application of preimplantation genetic diagnosis **(PGD)** is dependent on the ability to recover cells from an early embryo, accurately perform the genetic tests and produce a pregnancy without a significant loss in transfer success rate. In addition to sex determination, embryo biopsy can provide cells for detection of genes for inheritable diseases. Recent studies have shown that biopsy samples and blastocele fluid collected from equine embryos can be evaluated for sex and genetic diseases.

Summary

The foundation of equine embryo transfer has always been scientific research and future advancements in the field will also depend on research. Basic science, applied research, and retrospective studies from commercial breeding programs practices are all valuable in enhancing our knowledge of embryo biology and translation of laboratory techniques to clinical practice.

Suggested Reading

Allen WR, Wilshire S, Morris L, Crowhurst JS, Hillyer MH, Neal HH. Laparoscopic application of PGE$_2$ to re-establish oviductal patency and fertility in infertile mares: a preliminary study. Equine Vet J. 2006; 38: 454-459.

Carnevale EM. Oocyte transfer and gamete intrafallopian transfer in the mare. Animal Reproduction Science 2004; 82:617-624.

Hatzel JN, McCue PM, Ehrhart EJ, Charles JB, Ferris RA. Immunohistochemical localization of Early Pregnancy Factor (Hsp-10) in equine embryos. Journal of Equine Vet Science 2012: 32: 399.

Hinrichs K. Biopsy and vitrification of equine expanded blastocysts. Clinical Theriogenology 2011; 3:314-317.

Ohnuma K, Yokoo M, Kazuei I, Y Nambo, Miyake Y-I, Komatsu M, Takahashi J. Study of early pregnancy factor (EPF) in equine. American Journal of Reproductive Immunology 2000; 43:174-179.

Ortis HA, Foss RR, McCue PM, Bradecamp EA, Ferris RA, Hendrickson DA. Laparoscopic application of PGE2 to the oviductal surface enhances fertility in selected subfertile mares. J Equine Vet Science 2013; 33:896-900.

Squires EL, McCue PM. Superovulation. In: Equine Reproduction, Second Edition. McKinnon AO, Squiresm EL, Vaala WE and DD Varner DD (Eds). Wiley-Blackwell, West Sussex, United Kingdom pp. 1836-1845.

APPENDIX 1

EMBRYO TRANSFER SUPPLIES AND EQUIPMENT

Full Line of Embryo Transfer Products and Supplies

Bioniche Animal Health USA (Vétoquinol)
1615 NE Eastgate Blvd, Sec. H
Pullman, WA 99163
1-800-335-8595
www.bioniche.com

IMV International
11725 95th Ave. N.
Maple Grove, MN 55369
800-342-5468
www.imvusa.com

Minitube of America
PO Box 930187
Verona, WI 53593
800-646-4882
www.minitube.com

Veterinary Concepts, Inc.
P.O. Box 39
Spring Valley, WI 54767-0039
800-826-6948
www.veterinaryconcepts.com

Professional Embryo Transfer Supplies
PO Box 188
Canton, TX 75103-1088
800-634-2977
www.pets-inc.com

General Laboratory Supplies

Fisher Scientific
800-766-7000
www.fishersci.com

MWI
800-824-3703
www.mwivet.com

APPENDIX 2

FORMULARY FOR
EQUINE EMBRYO TRANSFER

Medication	Dosage, Route, Frequency	Indications
Altrenogest (2.2 mg/ml)	0.044 mg/kg. orally. q 24h	Suppression of behavioral estrus, synchronization of estrus, maintenance of pregnancy
Altrenogest (2.2 mg/ml)	0.088 mg/kg. orally. q 24h or 0.044 mg/kg. orally. q 12h (double dose)	Maintenance of pregnancy in high risk mares
Buserelin	10 to 50 μg. IM. q 6 h to 12h	GnRH agonist: stimulation of follicular development in anestrous, transitional or acyclic mares
Cloprostenol (250 μg/ml)	250 μg. IM. once	Termination of luteal activity, synchronization of estrus, termination of pregnancy, stimulation of uterine contractions (evacuation of uterine fluid): should not be administered in the early post-ovulation period due to adverse effects on development of the corpus luteum
Deslorelin (1.5 mg/ml)	1.5 mg. IM. once	Induction of ovulation
Deslorelin (low dose)	10 to 50 μg. IM. q 6h to q 12h	GnRH agonist: stimulation of follicular development in anestrous, transitional or acyclic mares
Dinoprost tromethamine (5 mg/ml)	10 mg. IM. once	Termination of luteal activity: synchronization of estrus, termination of pregnancy, stimulation of uterine contractions (evacuation of uterine fluid): should not be administered in the early post-ovulation period due to adverse effects on development of the corpus luteum

Drug	Dose	Indication
Estradiol (E_2)	5 to 10 mg, IM, q 24h	Stimulation of behavioral estrus in ovariectomized mares; used in conjunction with progesterone for estrous synchronization
Human Chorionic Gonadotropin (hCG) (10,000 units/vial)	1,500 to 3,000 units, IV or IM, once	Induction of ovulation
Oxytocin (20 IU/ml)	20 international units, IV or IM, q 6h to q 24h or as needed	Stimulation of uterine contractions (evacuation of uterine fluid), treatment of retained placenta, milk letdown
Progesterone-in-oil (P_4) (50mg/ml)	200mg, IM, q 24h	Maintenance of pregnancy
Progesterone-in-oil (P_4) (50 mg/ml)	150 mg, IM, q 24h	Suppression of behavioral estrus; synchronization of estrus and ovulation
Progesterone (long acting) (150 or 300 mg/ml)	1,500 mg, IM, q 7 days	Suppression of behavioral estrus, synchronization of estrus, maintenance of pregnancy
Progesterone/Estradiol (P&E) (50 mg P_4/3.3 mg E_2)	150 mg P4/10 mg E2, IM, q 24h	Synchronization of estrus, 'programming' time of ovulation in transitional mares, suppression of estrus
Prostaglandin E_1 (Misoprostol; Cytotec®) (100 µg/tablet)	1,000 to 2,000 µg, topically onto cervix, as needed	Cervical relaxation
Prostaglandin E_2 (0.2 mg/ml)	1.0 mls gel applied to surface of each oviduct	Applied to surface of oviducts via laparoscope to "unblock" oviducts suspected of luminal blockage with gelatinous masses that contain fibroblast cells

Miscellaneous Medications

Medication	Dosage, Route, Frequency	Indications
Acepromazine (Promace®) (10 mg/ml)	10 to 20 mg, IV, once	Sedation; relaxation of cervix prior to embryo transfer
Flunixin meglumine (50 mg/ml)	1.1 mg/kg, IV, once	Anti-inflammatory, antiprostaglandin; administered prior to transfer of an embryo; treatment of placentitis
Meclofenamic Acid	2.2 mg/kg, PO, q 12h	Prostaglandin inhibitor potentially used as adjunct therapy in embryo transfer
N-Butylscopolammonium (20 mg/ml)	0.08 – 0.12 mg/kg, IV (40 to 60 mg) administered 5 to 10 minutes prior to palpation	Relaxation of rectal musculature (decrease rectal pressure)
N-Butylscopolammonium Cream	Topical cream	Cervical relaxation
Propanetheline bromide	30 mg, IV, once	Rectal relaxation; wait 5 to 10 minutes after administration prior to palpation
Xylazine (100 mg/ml)	0.33 – 0.44 mg/kg, IV	Sedation; may be used prior to embryo transfer

Index

Printed and bound by CPI Group (UK) Ltd, Croydon, CR0 4YY

23/10/2024

01777696-0012